I0840922

The Truth About… Vol. 2 Vitamins
By B. K. Robinson
Copyright 2018© ALL RIGHTS RESERVED

Introduction
    I'm no doctor, nor do I have any kind of degree related to the subject matter of this book. As such you are welcome to judge me accordingly but, a whole lot of people have changed the world and the way you live and they did not have degrees either. So I recommend you read this booklet first, before you judge me and I think you will see that a person does not need a degree to be smart, hard working, well informed, and indeed an expert in their field.
    Although the horrendously overpriced rip-off colleges have not put me hundreds of thousands of dollars in debt, I am a consumer and I found myself looking down the massive vitamins and supplements aisle of a typical drug store and realized that there was absolutely no way a person could walk up, pick a multivitamin off the shelf, and get it right.
    Furthermore, I realized that there was no way anyone could pick ANY vitamin or supplement off of that shelf and get it right – that is, try to take something that would shore up what they perceive to be their weakness. And how could a person, like myself, even know what their weaknesses were in the first place?
    This series of books intends to address this problem. I have done all of the research and I can tell you exactly which products have the best ingredients – which ones work – and where appropriate, which ones have such useless ingredients that they are worth avoiding.
    And that's an important point, it is amazing to consider that some supplements on the very shelf I mentioned are almost completely useless, and it is amazing that they are even allowed to sell the garbage at all, but they are allowed to do it and we all know exactly why: greed and the insatiable thirst to steal that almighty dollar by the millions – the same greed, in the food industry that has made us all sick in the first place!
    If we all stop buying the poisons that the greedy monsters want to shove down our throats, then they will stop wasting their time manufacturing those cancer cocktails and maybe they might actually start making products that are good for us.
    One in three Americans will die of cancer, a disease that was one of the rarest known to medical science prior to World War II with only a handful – and I mean LESS THAN TEN – cases diagnosed by doctors each year. In the fifties these numbers exploded exponentially from hundreds per year to thousands to tens of thousands to hundreds of thousands of new cases each year. What changed? Two things: chemical additives to the foods we eat started appearing in the fifties and the nuclear bombs were

set off in the mid-forties through the fifties. These bombs create what we all know very well as the mushroom cloud, this thing sends radioactive fallout as high as 30 miles, that's the edge of space, and the upper atmospheric winds can distribute that fallout worldwide and it only takes ONE RADIOACTIVE ATOM to be absorbed by you, to ultimately possibly cause cancer in you.

We have no way of protecting ourselves from the radioactive fallout of these bombs or the Chernobyl and Fukushima disasters that have easily poured ten times the radioactive contamination into the Earth's atmosphere as all of the bombs before them did, but we can stop eating the POISONS that cause cancer and we can start eating the things that will make us healthier.

In the coming books I will not include the first chapter any more to save paper but the information in it is so important that I have to include it here at least a second time.

I would be remiss if I were to say that clinical trials and studies are the ultimate evidence for proving something: they are not. And I would seem to be a hypocrite if I quoted you one study and said there's the proof and then scoffed at the next study. What I will do is this: I will quote you studies that indicate "No negative outcome." For example, if a study showed that feeding people a massive overdose of some nutrient had no ill side effects, I will call that "conclusive evidence that the nutrient is safe." I will not quote a study that fed people a massive overdose and that then reported that the substance was toxic. The reason being that too much water is deadly (it is commonly known as drowning,) so these reports are not necessarily of value to us. I will report a study that shows the efficacy of a substance. For example, if a bunch of people are dying of beriberi, and they are given a massive vitamin B complex and return to health, then it stands to good reason that the vitamin B complex worked.

On the other hand I will not quote a study that indicates that something is not effective. The reason for this again is that the study is not necessarily conclusive. For example, giving a massive treatment of a nutrient to people dying of cancer does not mean that the treatment has no usefulness if all of the people died because: 1) We do not know what stage of the illness they were in (were they literally on their death beds already?) and 2) We do not know which particular cancer they had; there are roughly twelve major forms of cancer, you know a few of them like benign tumors versus malignant tumors, and tumors caused by a breakdown of the person's autoimmune system versus those caused by exposure to known cancer causing agents and so on. So some things might be highly effective against one kind and have no effect on another, but one thing is for certain: advising a person to stop consuming known toxins and to concentrate on eating healthy foods and taking vitamins and supplements, while it may not cure carcinomas, won't do any harm either.

Oh and one last thing before we begin: I am certain that almost every American who is not eating a solid well researched regimen of whole natural foods is MALNOURISHED. Three things are killing Americans:

1. They eat POISON in the form of CANCER CAUSING ADDITIVES to their PROCESSED foods on a DAILY BASIS. (And they are exposed to other POISONS also on a daily basis, like DIESEL ENGINE FUMES, HARSH CLEANER FUMES, etc.)
2. POOR DIET: even if you eat right, most of the plants are being grown in dead soil that has been overused for decades, the only reason the plants grow at all is because of the massive amounts of fertilizers being used on them – artificial, manufactured, chemical concoctions. This is what I affectionately call DIRTOPONICS. Just like HYDROPONICS or AEROPONICS, the plants must be given 100% of their nutritional requirements in order to grow, the only difference is that they are sitting in DEAD SOIL instead of pure water or air while they grow. Because of these conditions, many of the macro and micro-minerals are dramatically reduced or completely missing, having been absorbed completely out of the soil by crops decades ago. Even the current crops, manage to eek out an existence based on their fertilizer sources of nutrients but cannot possibly be producing the supplements we expect from them in the quantities that they should be producing, hence we are all malnourished even if we eat the right foods because they simply no longer contain adequate, or natural, levels of the nutrients that they should be providing us.
3. LACK OF EXERCISE: You cannot expect to be healthy if all you do is sit in your car on the way to work. Sit at a desk all day at work, and sit at your TV all evening when you get home. I talk about getting adequate EXERCISE in Volume 1.

This series is designed to guide you through the bewildering maze of the vitamin shelf at your favorite store and is not a substitute for professional advice. If you are currently on medication of any kind, you MUST CONSULT A DOCTOR before taking anything, including vitamins because they STRONGLY AFFECT the way your body works and can actually cause a VERY BAD REACTION in combination with certain strong medications.

Also I have aimed this series primarily at vitamins and minerals but they are ONLY THE BEGINNING, there are a multitude of ESSENTIAL NUTRIENTS (things you CANNOT SURVIVE WITHOUT) that are neither vitamins or minerals. These will be covered in an upcoming volume: The Truth About … MINERALS and ESSENTIAL NUTRIENTS.

Now, read and learn.

CHAPTER 1 – STOP EATING POISON

If you really want to be healthy, that is, if you are looking for the most effective vitamin/mineral/supplement, then you are interested in being healthy and staying healthy. And rule number one in working toward being healthy is to stop eating poison and to start eating foods that do not have a significant percentage of poison in their ingredients.

Now I cannot possibly list for you all of the poisons that the greedy moneygrubbers are putting into our foods – that would require far too much paper and make the book rather expensive, but I can give you a few examples and I think you'll get the idea and be able to identify poisons in your food with no trouble after that.

First a little chemistry, and I do mean a little. I'm no chemist, but I did study it in college and it was one of two possible choices for my major, the other was physics, but life and all of its problems, including health issues ultimately conspired to keep me from achieving my dreams. However, that was then, and this is now. And now that I have removed the greedy monsters from my life, a much healthier one now I might add, I can concentrate on bringing you the truth, not just about food, nutrients, and so on, but about everything.

Your stomach has one main function: to bathe everything that lands in it in a roughly pH 1 solution of Hydrochloric acid. This happens to be an incredibly dangerous and corrosive solution that while not as bad as alien blood (from the movie "Alien") it is one of the strongest acid solutions anywhere rivaling even the content of a car battery!

Anyway, the objective is to let that acid reduce complex molecules in the food into simpler ones and we're talking mainly about fats, starches and proteins all of which get cut down into smaller chunks, so starches are turned into sugars, proteins into amino acids and so on.

What is interesting about our stomach solution is that many things can dissolve in it, and if they dissolve in the solution, then it is also likely that they can be absorbed easily, either through the stomach lining itself which while unlikely is possible, but definitely through the intestinal walls and with great ease if the substance has been dissolved in the liquid released by the stomach into the beginning of the intestines called the duodenum. This section of intestine is tougher than the rest and can reabsorb the Hydrochloric acid that is still in the liquid called chyme (kyme) and get it out of there so it won't burn up the rest of your intestines.

Most, not all – we bear that in mind – Sodium salts will easily dissolve in the stomach acid. This frees the opposite piece in solution to be absorbed. For example, table salt is Sodium Chloride and it dissolves easily in the stomach solution yielding free Sodium ions and free Chloride ions. Both can be easily absorbed in the intestines thereafter. The Chloride ion is simply a Chlorine atom and you may have guessed from the nature of Hydrochloric acid, and the Mustard Gas used to kill thousands in World War 1 and the fact that adding it to your pool keeps microorganisms from infesting it, that this substance is abiotic or in layman's terms: it is a deadly poison to almost all forms of life.

Trust me, the fish in the sea have fought for millions of years just trying to stay alive while swimming through it – it is a POISON. And you do not need this poison in your body. Therefore, do not eat too much salt. Sodium by the way is not good for you in overabundance either.

Now remember, just about anything that starts with the name Sodium, Sodium blahblahblahate for example, is SOLUBLE in your stomach. And granted, you actually do need some sodium in your body, what the sports drink people say they give you to replenish your "electrolytes" but you don't need tons of it and potassium and magnesium may be by far the better "electrolytes" over sodium anyway. Also remember that just about anything like blahblahblahium Chloride is also very likely going to be SOLUBLE or EASILY absorbed and also free up the POISON known as CHLORINE. Again, you need a little, so your stomach can actually manufacture the HydroCHLORIC acid it uses to continue your digestive process, but again, you don't need tons of this poison inside of you. Where does the excess of these things go anyway? Straight into the liver.

That's where every single molecule you eat goes by the way, through what the health professionals call affectionately, the HEPATIC PORTAL VEIN. Basically all of the capillaries in the walls of your intestines that are absorbing every molecule of what you ate gather back together into a big vein that feeds directly into your liver. This organ gets the first look at what you had for dinner, every time. This is how what you had for dinner gets regulated. Otherwise you would have dinner, say a steak and a potato, and the potato would be converted into sugars which would hit your bloodstream within an half an hour and you'd be on the same sugar rush as if you had bolted down a two liter bottle of soda – that would not be a very good plan, and so that's why everything funnels into the liver.

The liver will grab up almost everything and then try to slowly release it back into the bloodstream over the next several hours, at least. And in the case of POISONS it does recognize an amazing number of them and tries to permanently take them out of circulation. You can bet it regulates the electrolytes since a particularly salty meal would likely cause you to have a heart attack if it didn't (the electrolytes are involved in the electrical field of the entire human body – subject for a coming book – and dramatically affect the heart which does have a natural pacemaker by the way.) And you can bet it does everything it can, including letting its own cells DIE for the cause, in trying to remove POISONS from the stream coming from the intestines and you can bet that one of these is CHLORINE.

Now the liver can take some abuse along these lines and regenerate on its own, that is its job, but pushing it to its limits and beyond every single day leads to liver disease, liver failure, cirrhosis of the liver (too many cells have been killed repeatedly to the point where it can't grow back as fast as it is being destroyed by the POISON known as ETHANOL – usually – and so the liver literally dies a long slow horrible death and takes the overindulgent drunken idiot through a similar long slow and horrible death along with it.) Yes, you guessed correctly, ETHANOL, the alcohol in alcoholic beverages is one of the worst POISONS you can pickle your liver in – 4 to 6 ounces of alcohol (13% or less) in one sitting one time per day is acceptable for healthy individuals only. Any more than that and you are taxing your liver unnecessarily and that will come back to KILL YOU in the long run.

Ok, so what do we know? Sodium blahblahblahate and blahblahblahium Chloride are both likely very SOLUBLE in our digestive tracts but they will dump unwanted POISONS in the form of excess sodium ions, which the liver will try to regulate, but in the end will release into your blood and remember these are electrolytes and they can really mess up your electrical field and mess with your HEART which is why all the doctors scream – no salt – and the other extremely toxic one CHLORINE which is why they pump the tap water with a fraction of a percent of it which is good enough to kill just about every known microbe on Earth. Microbes are nothing more than single celled organisms … cells … cells that DIE when even a TRACE of CHLORINE is around. Oh yeah, you happen to be made out of cells … cells that die in the presence of chlorine – get it?

Now let's look at a few food label ingredient items shall we? I won't mention the actual food products I found these in, for fear of being mercilessly sued into dust by the greedy money worshipping owners of the companies that manufacture these beautifully packaged POISONS. Here are some of my favorite HORRORS that I have found in food – that you EAT:

1) SODIUM BENZOATE – This may be in every single packaged food product on Earth, or at least in the United States, as a "preservative." Well, it might keep the food the same color and texture for a longer period of time, but it is certainly not preserving the person who eats it. Case in point: Benzene, (the Benzoate ion simply has an oxygen atom bonded to it, which does help lessen its TOXICITY but it certainly does not make it into manna from heaven either) used to be found in every high school chemistry lab in the United States, including my own many years ago. But you won't find it there any more. Why? Because a lab did a study and

found that the vapors (it is highly volatile with a unique aroma.
Another such small organic molecule with a strange unique aroma
is Napthalene or moth balls) and those fumes are extremely
carcinogenic and we can't have the children being exposed to
them can we? Absolutely not! But make sure they get their daily
DOSE OF THE POISON in the meals they eat EVERY SINGLE
DAY! Even if Sodium Benzoate's ion is 1/10,000th the carcinogen
as the precursor Benzene, the fact is that every single man,
woman and child in the United States eats this POISON almost on
a DAILY BASIS. And the last time I checked 300 million divided by
ten thousand is still 30,000; as in cases of CANCER. I don't want
to be one of them, do you?
2) SODIUM CASEINATE – This is one of my favorites. Ever hear
of Casein paint? Basically this food product had wall paint in it and
the manufacturer had the audacity to put in parenthesis an
explanation for why this ingredient was in the food: "added for
texture." They added this garbage – house paint! – to give the food
the right TEXTURE. Personally, I think I stopped wanting to eat
paint by the time I reached the age of two years old, but thanks
anyway.
3) SODIUM STEARATE – Another favorite, this is SOAP. Now I
admit I've got quite the potty mouth, but my mother never washed
my mouth out with soap, and as an adult I am not about to start
either. These monsters didn't even have the decency to explain to
me why they put the soap into my food either. Well I guess it
keeps it clean right? Ever wonder why soap cleans so well? It
bonds with fats and oils and is also soluble in water, this means
that it grabs up the oils and dissolves with them into the water and
then rinses away squeaky clean. Well I don't want all of my cells
which are little bags of water and OIL to get rinsed away leaving
my bones squeaky clean … I'd like to keep all of my cells right
there where they are! This stuff is appearing in vitamin pills like
crazy as Magnesium Stearate. It is almost impossible to find a pill
that does NOT have it. Personally I don't want to swallow a small
chunk of soap, but it looks like they are giving us little choice in the
matter.
4) YELLOW #5 – This is a particular pet peeve of mine. This well
known carcinogen – and I mean there are plenty of studies
explicitly showing this nuisance to be a verifiable cancer causing
killer – is in almost as many things as that confounded menace
Sodium Benzoate. This garbage causes cancer. Do not eat
anything containing it and the manufacturers will eventually get the
idea and stop using it.
5) The six major SUGAR SUBSTITUTES – acesulfame potassium,
aspartame, neotame, sacharrin, sucralose, and sorbitol. I cannot
speak for all of them but I can speak for some of them in particular.
Saccharin is a well known cancer causing TOXIN, in fact it makes
an excellent rat poison and roach killer. Personally anything that

can kill a roach is nothing I want to be eating, these are the critters that can eat book binding glue – get it? Aspartame has some studies linking it to cancer and so does sucralose. I think you're getting the idea: I'd rather risk rotting my teeth than dying of cancer. Now I know the diabetics are in trouble, they can't just go back to sugar. But that's ok, there are natural sugar substitutes and in their case they may have to consult with a doctor to see which ones will not mess with their blood sugar counts. As for the rest of us, do not bother consuming any artificial sweeteners, they cause cancer, period.

Now that you have several examples of additives to your food, what do they all have in common? They sound like they belong on the shelf of a college chemistry laboratory and NOT IN YOUR FOOD. And if it seems that way, if it sounds like that's the way it should be (those mad scientists experiments should be on the shelf of a lab somewhere, and not in your food) then chances are YOU'RE RIGHT. So read the label and if it contains anything I listed above, then it is automatically OUT, and if it has some other SODIUM blahblahblahATE or blahblahblahIUM blahATE in it – then DON'T EAT IT!

I guarantee you this: if the food product has an ingredients label, and is in a cardboard or plastic wrapped package then it has at least one of these manmade, manufactured CHEMICALS in it, and if man made it, it is thousands of times more likely to be POISONOUS, than if nature made it – even the same "exact" molecule and I'll tell you why right now.

No human being has ever SEEN an atom. There is evidence that they exist and I am not trying to deny that, what I am saying is that no one has ever gotten all the way down there to get a really good close up look at one. So there may be minute differences between one atom and another, in fact quantum theory confirms that, and there may be extremely subtle differences between two allegedly identical molecules, one made in a lab and the other made in a tree. There is scientific proof for this statement as well: sugar. You have heard of "left-handed" sugar before, right? It means that the molecule is large and extended in three dimensions like a shoe, it has length, width and height and a recognizable top side and bottom side and a characteristic, like the top view shape or bend in the shoe that makes the left one unique from the right one, and you can't just turn it over and use it, because your foot can't go through the bottom of the shoe in order to put it on. In other words, the left shoe and the right shoe are unique and cannot be interchanged; you will never want to buy a pair of shoes in which there were two left shoes in it, unless you actually have two left feet, of course.

The same is true of the three dimensional shape of the sugar molecule and interestingly enough, all plants manufacture right handed sugar and they do not manufacture any left handed sugar.

And in a laboratory, starting with say, carbon dioxide, and water (just like the plants do) humans could manufacture sugar, but without a differentiating enzyme they would make 50% right handed sugar and 50% left handed sugar. The differentiating enzyme would be any substance used in the process of manufacturing the sugar that itself had only right handed molecules in it, that could then control the outcome and make all of the resultant molecules left or right handed. Whew!

One more statement concerning that: since we can't make exclusively right or left handed molecules from scratch (starting with molecules that do not have left or right handedness to them) then that differentiating enzyme would have to be collected from a living thing, because life is the only thing that can make exclusively rught-handed molecules and has been doing this for eons. Since WE are living things and therefore WE have a lot of exclusively left or right handed molecules in our construction and cellular processes, then it makes sense that at some point, if we encounter a quantity of the "wrong way" molecule, that it won't just be useless, but it might very well be POISONOUS to us as well. And there are such examples known to science, where the right handed one is good for us and the left handed one is bad for us.

Now I have had a rather lengthy excursion into this subject of left and right handed molecules and chemists call any molecule that has a sufficiently complex three dimensional shape that it can have left and right handed molecules "stereoenantiomers" (YIKES! But now you've got yourself a nice $50 word to throw around at your friends!) And now I can return to my original point, there is no way for us to know all of the subtleties within molecules containing even five atoms, let alone dozens or hundreds and many molecules involved in nutrition are huge. Therefore, manmade, synthetic, artificial, whatever you want to call them, versions of molecules are not necessarily the SAME EXACT MOLECULES and can therefore be subtly different in such a way that they are SETTING YOU UP FOR DEATH, likely in the form of CANCER, and at the very least ARE HIGHLY INEFFECTIVE in the case of MANUFACTURED VITAMINS.

So what should you buy? Even if we cannot tell if the vitamins are from natural sources or if they have been manufactured, we can at least tell the difference between, USABLE FORMS and forms that are not so readily absorbed and used by the body.

Go to the produce section of your favorite grocery store and buy some fresh vegetables and fruits. Yes, they are all saturated in insecticides and fungicides and fertilizers and so on. But there is no stopping that unless you grow your own which I highly recommend by the way, or unless you pay plenty more to get "organic" produce. I'll discuss "organic" produce in an upcoming book too. Still, I'll side with the foods NOT BATHED IN SODIUM BENZOATE, SACCHARIN, and YELLOW #5 than those that are.

Incidentally, I have found at least one food product that had ALL THREE of those in it. I am amazed that people don't fall to the floor, cold and hard, while partaking of that CANCER COCKTAIL.

What else can you eat? Go to the meats section and get yourself some chicken, or some fish. I often grab a pack of pork chops when they are on sale. Contrary to popular belief, as long as you cook it well, it won't do any more harm to you in moderation than any other NATURAL thing made by the EARTH as opposed to those things manufactured by some greedy monster. It will certainly do far less harm to me than that little pink packet in your coffee.

Check the labels. Some brands might add things you don't want. If the chicken looks too yellow, guess what they have bathed it in? Yellow #5, you got it! Incidentally when I indict that garbage I am referring to ALL artificial food colorings and flavors, not just that specific one. Don't eat that POISON.

Yes, I know that most artificial flavorings are chemically "identical" to the real ones found in nature, but why is it that artificial grape flavored things taste nothing like natural grape flavored things? How identical are they? I believe I already warned you about this (sort of the same molecule not being exactly the same) and frankly I do not know how identical these molecules are to the natural ones, and I guarantee you that the greedy monsters POISONING YOUR FOOD with it don't know any more about it than the greatest physicists and chemists on Earth who would neither confirm nor deny my claims with anything more substantial than the Heisenberg Uncertainty principle, which supports my claim that they are different just as much as it would support their claim that undetectable differences are irrelevant. Sorry for the rant, but this stuff is KILLING US and if I get going down hill, there's no stopping me. The bad news is that the greedy monsters putting this manufactured POISONOUS CANCER CAUSING garbage into our food DON'T CARE EITHER. "Just sit down, shut up, buy it and eat it."

On rare occasion I buy canned goods and I do buy them for the purposes of having an emergency store of food, just in case the world ends tomorrow. I buy "No Salt" versions whenever possible and I buy one can and go home and open it. If the can is LINED, and not simply the raw metal, then I'll go back and get the twenty cans or whatever I intend to get. Even the canneries have figured out that when their food tastes like the can, people will go for the other product with the LINING in their cans so that their food does not taste like the can: and so most of them line the cans with an inert material like a thin plastic coating. It costs more to manufacture the cans than just making the cans without the lining so why do you think they bother doing it? Because WE THE CONSUMERS HAVE SPOKEN WITH OUR WALLETS on the subject and that is exactly what we can always do and make these monsters STOP POISONING OUR FOOD.

Back to the discussion, if the cans are lined then I buy the stuff. If the can is NOT lined, then very likely the contents do taste like the can, do not even give that stuff to the dog, throw it away and I'll tell you why.

It's called metal poisoning. You know, the thousands of dollars you have to spend for a licensed contractor to come in and strip your walls of lead based paint and repaint your house so you can actually sell it on the open market. Now, luckily the monsters that have elected themselves to be the ones to feed us all, have found cheaper metals than lead to put our food into or trust me they would do it. Still those metals are not necessarily better for you than lead either. And the one I am talking about in particular is aluminum. There are reports that this may be related to Alzheimer's Disease; another very rare illness that has now magically become a massive epidemic. Where did this thing come from? Aluminum cans, especially aluminum soda pop cans. This is the perfect storm: aluminum in contact with a weak acid, Carbonic Acid, which in solution can form a strong base and suddenly grab up the aluminum molecules in the walls of the can and take them into solution as Aluminum Carbonate: not necessarily tons of this, just a minuscule trace amount, but what if this garbage gets inside you and somehow gets trapped in your brain chemistry and NEVER GOES AWAY? Then tomorrow you suck down another pop, then another, and eventually, from accumulating the POISON over decades in your brain, you don't recognize yourself in the mirror any more. STAY AWAY FROM ANY HIGHLY ACIDIC substance in any UNLINED METAL CONTAINER. That would mean any fruit product in particular. Do I buy canned fruits? Yes I do, some of them come in unlined cans, and they hit the trash can and I make a note of the product so I will never buy it again in life.

I have a gallery of photos on my computer to remind me of what products have been designed to kill me so that I will never buy them again. I would love to share, but with all those foaming mouthed billionaire bastards lurking out there, who would slowly lower their own mothers into the pits of hell just to make a nickel, I don't know if I would SURVIVE long enough to be sued.

Now take a moment to consider the following: how long would you survive without air, in particular oxygen? A few minutes at most. We could therefore say correctly that gaseous oxygen is the ultimate and most essential of all nutrients. Without it a human body shuts down and dies within minutes. This is because the oxygen provides the "oxidizer" for our cells to burn fuel (sugars mostly) from which they derive the energy to function. No energy to function, means no life and the main organ that has by far the highest demand for oxygen is the brain and that's exactly why you die so fast without air, because your brain, properly functioning, is that which is conscious and is in essence you. It is fascinating to note that most of the rest of the body can get along quite well for extended periods of time without oxygen, but that is of no use when the brain, which is the person, dies so fast without it.

Now our respiration, our breathing, which provides this most essential of all nutrients, only needs to take up oxygen (and get rid of built up Carbon Dioxide which is the result of the metabolic burning of the sugars in our cells) and nothing else; a very simple bodily function and requirement.

The point I am driving at here, is that although the process of eating is not as imperative as breathing, in that you will not starve to death in minutes if you stop (although some people eat as if they think they will) this does not change the fact that if you do stop eating, that you will die. Therefore eating is an imperative process, as imperative as breathing, even though the time delay between stopping it is much more protracted, the outcome is the same.

The major difference is that eating which involves the consumption into the digestive tract of essential nutrients, is the opposite of the simplicity of breathing, in which we do it to take up one simple nutrient. In eating, we absorb gigantic collections of gigantic molecules in such profusions and complexities that we may never be able to fully analyze a complete and healthy natural diet consisting of fruits, vegetables, and animal products.

But although we may not be able to fully chemically analyze our nutritional needs, that does not mean that those needs do not exist and it does not mean that we should just throw our hands up and give up. All that this means is that the mad scientists will never be able to provide us with a George Jetson diet of nothing but completely artificially manufactured pills that will keep us healthy for a long lifespan.

What I ultimately want to convince you of, with this argument is that:

1. There can never be an adequate substitution for natural foods. You can certainly take a Vitamin A pill to make sure that you get enough each day, but carrots contain not only all the Vitamin A that you need, but they contain beta-carotene which is a powerful anti-oxidant that helps defend your entire body and all of its cells from being damaged by free radicals or "oxidants" but this exact same substance can be easily converted by the body into more Vitamin A as needed: that's why I would recommend to anyone concerned about Vitamin A to eat carrots, as many as you can choke down, it is very unlikely to overdose on beta-carotene although you CAN overdose on pure Vitamin A.

2. By eating natural foods you will take in nutrients that no one even knows exist, but the human body needs them nevertheless. The more variety you have in your natural food

diet, the more likely you are to take in something that your body actually desperately needs.

3. Cravings have been suspected for years to involve a method by which the body reports a serious deficiency to the brain, and the craving is the way in which the brain drives the person to get the missing nutrient. Listen to your cravings and more importantly, keep rotating and changing your diet from one day to the next so that you never fall short for more than five days in a row of anything your body might need.

4. We know that all of our food, especially in the developed countries, from the plants, fruits, vegetables, grains, to the livestock that feeds on these plants are seriously lacking in critical nutrients because of the long dead dirt in which they have been cultivated. But the grape still looks like a grape, so it has still been able to construct its cells in all of their amazing complexity despite these shortcomings and therefore it has constructed complex molecules, that the mad scientists still have yet to discover or understand, and that your body needs in order to survive and to thrive. So despite my warnings that the plants and animals we eat are deficient, that does not mean that they are devoid of nutritional value. You must eat as many all-natural items in as much variety as you can in order to maintain optimal health and you must avoid at all costs all manufactured and processed foods because they are rife with cancer causing poisons and the processing has destroyed most if not all of the potential nutrients in them.

Nothing from the Earth will give you cancer. Yes there are a few naturally occurring substances that can give you cancer but usually only when WE PROCESS them into products which then cause us to be OVEREXPOSED to them. And yes, there are many poisonous plants, especially berries. I always wondered why the plants would make poisonous fruit. After all, their goal is to get something to come along and eat them so that the something will wander off and spread the seeds (this is the goal of all edible fruit by the way.) And the reason that so many berries are poisonous is that the plant does not want US to eat the fruit, it wants the birds to eat the berries. Many berries that are poisonous to us are not so to the birds. And they are FAR BETTER seed spreaders than we are since some of them migrate thousands of miles and the berry seeds can pass clean through the bird's digestive tract unscathed and end up in another state (probably on my windshield.)

The point is that we know what's poisonous in nature and we simply avoid all of those things. But we do not know what is manmade and poisonous in our food, other than the fact that most of those artificial additives eventually turn out to be toxic. The best plan is to err on the side of caution and stop eating anything that has manufactured chemicals in it.

But the Tomato doesn't have a Nutrition Label, how do I make sure I get my daily recommended dose of vitamins, minerals, and other supplements? The simple answer: you will never know. But I better explain that statement. The FDA's Recommended Daily Allowance or RDA of nutrient "requirements" should say "MINIMUM recommended daily allowance of REQUIREMENTS" since without them you will get sick and die. These values were mostly established back in the early 20th century with the discoveries of such things as vitamins and so on. For example, the FDA's Recommended Daily Allowance for Vitamin C is 60mg. This might keep you from getting scurvy and dying, but it is nowhere near what a person really needs to stay at the OPTIMUM of health and there is a significant difference between bare minimum survival versus THRIVE-LEVEL for maintaining optimum health.

Everyone knows that Vitamin C can help keep you from catching a cold and it can help you get over one quicker, so we all know that it works with the immune system somehow. Incidentally the "professionals" all insist that there is no clinical evidence showing that Vitamin C helps to prevent you from catching colds or from getting sick. This is what I call RIDICULOUS. If one hundred people purposely limit themselves to 60mg of Vitamin C per day I will bet you whatever QUANTITY of MONEY you feel like LOSING that more of them will get a cold of some degree during the next year than another group if they all take 1000mg (or better 2 to 3 thousand mg per day.) And I will bet you all of the MONEY YOU JUST PAID ME from LOSING the previous year's bet that far FEWER of the 60mg/day people will get sick in the subsequent year if they go up to 1000mg/day, so be careful because I plan on taking a LOT OF YOUR MONEY ON THIS BET. And while taking 60mg per day they might not die of scurvy but they will only be BARELY SURVIVING and will certainly not be THRIVING and will spend their lives in POOR OVERALL HEALTH until they raise that VITAMIN C daily intake up to THRIVE-LEVEL.

Vitamin C is a "safe" vitamin. And what I mean by that is that you cannot overdose on it (I suppose if you bought a 100 count bottle of 1000mg tablets and took them all in one sitting… you'd probably vomit them all back up and that would serve you right.) It is water soluble, which is part of the reason why you can't overdose on it because your body will eliminate any excess quantity in the urine. Interestingly enough it is highly pungent and easily detected in the urine and I have consumed as many as 3,000mg in a day and my body has never "thrown out" any noticeable excess. Cats make their own Vitamin C, by the way, and those little creatures produce thousands of milligrams of it per day to support those little bodies. We are significantly larger and should therefore need significantly more than they do. Incidentally we lost the ability to make our own Vitamin C when our ancestors discovered that oranges tasted good, and we've been dependent on fruits to get it ever since.

My point here is that most of the recommended minimum daily requirements as posted on those food labels are either ridiculous because they are based on amounts established in experiments conducted over fifty years ago designed to find out where the threshold was between surviving and dying – NOT the threshold between THRIVING and living a LONG and HEALTHY life versus barely hanging on in misery and poor health. Or they are meaningless because they are the average numbers for the herd, and the last time I checked, I am not an average member of the human herd; I do not have 2.4 children, make $30,000 a year, or stand 5'11" tall. And I am very willing to bet that I do not have the same nutritional requirements as the average person who has 2.4 children, makes $30,000 a year and stands 5'11" tall either.

So let's take a look at this situation. Here are the FDA's (Minimum) Recommended Daily Allowances for those nutrients for which they have established a baseline and bear in mind that there are many nutrients for which they have no idea what the baseline minimum daily requirement for them should be:

FDA's Minimum RDA Requirements of the Vitamins

Name	A.K.A.s (Forms)	100% RDA
Vitamin A	Retinol, Retinal	5000 IU (1)
	Beta-Carotene	5000 IU (1)
	Retinoic acid	NAN (0)
Vitamin B1	Thiamine	1.5mg
Vitamin B2	Riboflavin	1.7mg
Vitamin B3	Niacin, Niacinamide	20mg
Vitamin B5	Pantothenic acid	10mg
Vitamin B6	Pyridoxine, pyridoxal, and pyridoxamine.	2mg
Vitamin B7	Biotin	300mcg
Vitamin B9	Folic acid, "Folate"	400mcg
Vitamin B12	n-cobalamin (See Description below)	6mcg(2)
Choline	phosphatidycholine	550mg
Vitamin C	L-Ascorbic acid	60mg (3)
Vitamin D3	cholecalciferol	400 IU
Vitamin E	x-tocopherol	30 IU (4)
Vitamin K	Menaquinone, phylloquinone	80mcg

(0) NAN, Not A Nutrient, under normal circumstances you do not need to take this form.

(1) 1 IU is the biological equivalent of 0.3 mcg retinol, or of 0.6 mcg beta-carotene in the USA, and in Canada. A 50/50

mixture of 5000IU would therefore contain 750.0 mcg retinol and 1500 mcg beta-carotene.
(2) This is a very small amount, (6 micrograms) and the different forms may require quite different values
(3) This is a very small RDA but the essential nutrients with these tiny RDA's are still vital.
(4) 1 IU of Vitamin E is the biological equivalent of about 0.667mg d-alpha-tocopherol or of 1 mg of dl-alpha-tocopherol acetate. (yes, they sound like chemistry lab chemicals, I know!)

It should be noted that there are many more nutrients for which the FDA has not established a Recommended Daily Allowance yet. These include but are certainly not limited to: Boron, Silicon, Vanadium, Nickel, Tin, flavinoids, phytosterols, etc. NOTE: Nickel is a known irritant and allergen. Be very careful when selecting multivitamins that contain it.

And we have only just begun! There are nutrients that are still completely undiscovered. How do I know that? Because they are being discovered all the time and no one knows the complete composition and architecture of a single living cell, and humans have trillions upon trillions of them and so do the REAL foods that you eat.

Now some of these supplements are not as safe as Vitamin C. Vitamin A for example is quite dangerous. You can overdose on it and it can mess you up if you do that. This is because it is oil soluble, but not water soluble making it much more difficult to eliminate should you overdose on it and believe me, you can. I did and it is not the kind of experience you want to go through twice, trust me. (I was on medication for severe acne, and one of the programs that I tried was oral and topical Vitamin A combined, my doctor took me off of that within a week when he saw the reaction I had.)

So what we really need to know is which ones are the "safe" ones, that we can pig out on (sort of) and which ones we better take it easy with (bad grammar, ending a sentence with a preposition, I know, but I consider this book a conversation between me and all of my good friends much more than a go for the Pulitzer.) It would also be extremely helpful if we knew what each nutrient offers us so we can pick and choose where we want to pile on heavy and where we might go ahead and stick with the long standing norms listed by the FDA (at least we can be certain that they are not excesses that could cause us trouble.)

That's exactly what this series is all about.

END OF CHAPTER QUIZ
1. The weight of an IU (International Unit) is the same for all nutrients (i.e. 1 IU of one vitamin weighs the same as 1 IU of another) True or False?

ANSWER: False. The IU for a particular nutrient has been established for it independently. An IU for one nutrient may be significantly different in weight from another.

2. Vitamins are:
    A. Chemicals (naturally occurring)
    B. Elements (single atoms of a single element such as Boron)
    C. Neither A or B
    D. Both A and B

    ANSWER: A. Naturally occurring chemicals. The minerals are elements, although their usable forms are usually compounds, or chemicals, as well.

3. The only nutrients you need to worry about are vitamins and minerals. True or False?

    ANSWER: False. There are many known essential nutrients that are technically not minerals or vitamins. The Omega-3 fatty acids, found in abundance in most fish are an example.

4. Vitamins each exist in one form. True of False?

    ANSWER: False. This is one of the most confusing things about nutrients; many exist in many different forms and some forms are significantly different from others and we cannot be sure that the form found in nature that is extracted from a natural source is chemically identical to a synthesized one manufactured in a laboratory even if the mad scientists insist that it is.

6. At the very least all vitamins (and the other essential nutrients) should be acquired daily:

    A. In their natural whole food sources
    B. In at the very least 100% of the RDA amounts
    C. A variety of natural food sources as much as possible
    D. All of the above

    Answer: D. All of the above. A diet consisting of no processed packaged foods and well chosen whole natural foods will go a long way toward ending chronic deficiencies of virtually ALL 41 known essential nutrients that the body MUST have on a daily basis. Varying our whole natural foods diet ensures that you will get many unknown nutrients your body needs as well.

7. In emergencies or if you simply can't find the whole food that will satisfy your daily requirement of any particular vitamin the best recourse would be:

    A. Just skip it
    B. Get any over the counter supplement
    C. Double it tomorrow in some superfood.
    D. Get it in a high quality natural source supplement

    Answer: D. If you can't find the foods that contain the vitamin or any other essential nutrient, do not settle for store bought low quality supplements; shop for high quality natural source products instead.

I'll get straight to it here, but I do want to make a blanket statement concerning all of the following nutrients: whatever it is that we BELIEVE they do for us, it is very likely that they participate much more deeply in the human body than anyone suspects and without them you will indeed die sooner than you should, and you will be miserable and sick all the way to your early and bitter end, so find them and take them. The following chapters will deal with which forms are the best and which products are the best ones to take and which FOODS are LOADED with them.

This listing is set up numbering each major nutrient and then listing their ALTERNATE FORMS below them in the lettered entries below each nutrient.

1. **VITAMIN A:** linked to eye health, specifically the proper function of the retina. It is also linked to skin health. Deficiency of Vitamin A can lead to loss of vision and ultimately even blindness as well as bad skin rashes and chronic disorders of the skin. Vitamin A is also light sensitive and breaks down in light and should be kept in a cold, dark environment.[1]

   A. beta-carotene: naturally occurring in large quantities in carrots, basically the molecule consists of two Vitamin A molecules linked together. This form is non-toxic, in fact it is an ANTIOXIDANT which means it helps to ERADICATE TOXINS. This means you can eat a lot of carrots, and it is far safer than popping manufactured Vitamin A pills.

   B. Retinoic Acid – used as a topical treatment for skin disorders this is a non-reversible form that your body cannot metabolize back into straight Vitamin A and does not have the usefulness to the body that Vitamin A does.

2. **VITAMIN B:** Once thought to be a single Vitamin, there turned out to be eight of them. Their functions are sundry and suffice it to say that if you fall short in any one of the "B Complex" you probably won't live very long. The B vitamins are mostly water soluble and relatively safe to take in moderate excess. I would rather have too much of the B vitamins than not enough.

   A. **VITAMIN B1:** a.k.a. Thiamine, the sulfur containing vitamin is linked to proper brain and nervous system function. Its derivatives are linked to a variety of cellular processes as well. Deficiency causes a disease called beriberi affecting the nervous system and is generally rather nasty and it will kill you if you don't come into some thiamine before it's too late. In non-fatal deficiency, symptoms may include: malaise, weight loss, irritability and confusion.[2]

   B. **VITAMIN B2:** a.k.a. Riboflavin, like thiamine, riboflavin is linked to a wide variety of cellular processes. Deficiency leads to: cracked and red lips, inflammation of the lining of the mouth and tongue, mouth ulcers, cracks at the corners of the mouth, sore throat, dry and scaling skin, fluid in the mucous membranes, iron-deficiency anemia, and the eyes may also become bloodshot, itchy, watery and sensitive to bright light. Riboflavin is bright yellow and relatively non-soluble in water. Humans continuously dump riboflavin in the urine and overindulgence will lead to extremely bright yellow urine, but even in extended trials with doses in excess of 400,000mg per day clinicians still reported no adverse side effects.[3]

C. **VITAMIN B3:** a.k.a. Niacin and Niacinamide. Mild deficiency symptoms include: slow metabolism, decreased tolerance to cold. Severe deficiency of niacin results in the disease pellagra. Symptoms include: diarrhea, dermatitis, dementia, lesions on the lower neck, darkening of the skin, thickening of the skin, inflammation of the mouth and tongue, digestive disturbances, amnesia, delirium, and eventually death. Psychiatric symptoms of niacin deficiency include: irritability, poor concentration, anxiety, fatigue, restlessness, apathy, and depression. Niacin blocks the production of LDL, the "bad" cholesterol, and promotes the increase of HDL, the "good" cholesterol. One might say that Niacin deficiency gives you the ultimate high cholesterol form of death. Take it, but settle in at no more than 35mg/day. Niacin can cause an effect known as "flushing" basically a skin rash accompanied by a prickly sensation. Reduce your intake if you experience this. Alternate form: Tryptophan: the liver can make niacin and it is assumed that a healthy person will make all that they need. 60mg of tryptophan (an amino acid in all proteins) is needed to make 1mg of niacin. Vitamin B6 and iron are also needed.[4]

D. **VITAMIN B5:** a.k.a. Pantothenic acid. Required in order to synthesize coenzyme-A (CoA), as well as to synthesize and metabolize proteins, carbohydrates, and fats. Deficiency disease is extremely rare because this nutrient is found in almost all foods, but symptoms of low CoA levels include: impaired energy production, irritability, fatigue, and apathy. Acetylcholine synthesis is also impaired; so neurological symptoms can also appear including numbness, and muscle cramps. Deficiency can also cause hypoglycemia, or an increased sensitivity to insulin. Symptoms of deficiency are typical of deficiency in most B vitamins: restlessness, malaise, sleep disturbances, nausea, vomiting, and abdominal cramps.[5] Alternate forms: Calcium pantothenate. Yes, this is a chemistry name, but trust me a lot of these nutrients have been analyzed and their chemistries are very well understood and they will have such names. If I say it's OK, while I am going ballistic about chemistry names, then it is OK. This form is actually easier to absorb because it is a salt, but remember that it is bringing calcium with it, so don't find yourself taking too much calcium unless you want to grow a snail shell around yourself. And also remember that there is a difference between MANUFACTURED chemicals and those EXTRACTED from NATURAL SOURCES and getting all of your essential nutrients from whole natural foods is HIGHLY PREFERRED. We'll deal with this is upcoming chapters.

E. **VITAMIN B6:** occurs in three forms: pyridoxine (a.k.a. pyridoxine hydrochloride), pyridoxal, and pyridoxamine. A typical B vitamin related to many cellular functions including: the balancing of sodium and potassium, promoting red blood cell production, linked to cardiovascular health by decreasing the formation of homocysteine, balancing hormonal changes in women and assists the immune system. B6 can be toxic in extremely high doses (10 times the RDA) but should be safe at values closer to the RDA. It is used in the production of the brain neurotransmitters serotonin, dopamine, norepinephrine and epinephrine. Deficiency of pyridoxine can cause anemia, nerve damage, seizures, skin problems, and sores in the mouth. Like all B vitamins, it should be a priority.[6]

F. **VITAMIN B7:** a.k.a. Biotin. This vitamin is a coenzyme in the metabolism of fatty acids and leucine and like all B vitamins it plays a vast and complicated set of roles in cellular processes. Biotin is a water soluble vitamin that clinical studies have shown to be one of the few with little to any toxicity even in grossly exaggerated proportions. Deficiency disease is most likely caused by eating too many raw egg whites (and almost nothing else can cause it) but that doesn't make eggs the evil everyone wants to make them out to be either. Cooking the egg white neutralizes the chemistry that strongly binds to biotin and makes eating eggs not only safe, but one of the best sources of many nutrients including the B vitamins! Symptoms include: hair loss, conjunctivitis, a scaly red rash around the eyes, nose, mouth and genital area, depression, lethargy, hallucination, and numbness and tingling of the extremities. A very characteristic facial rash, together with an unusual facial fat distribution, has been called the "biotin-deficient face" by some medical experts.[7]

G. **VITAMIN B9:** a.k.a. Folic acid. Typical B vitamin with sundry cellular functional roles, including: synthesis of DNA, repairing DNA, and methylation of DNA. It is especially important in aiding rapid cell division and growth. There are clinical trials that indicate that it "feeds cancer" but that is only because cancer cells like all other cells multiply, they just multiply "out of control" because their DNA has been damaged. Note that Folic acid FIXES DNA and I would argue that someone who already had cancer could possibly feed the cancer by suddenly taking a train load of B9, but the benefits outweigh the risks and I would bet that B9 will do more REPAIR and PREVENTION of cancer than it will to feed it. Nevertheless, those already diagnosed with cancer should consult a doctor about taking B9 for these obvious reasons. Deficiency symptoms include diarrhea, macrocytic anemia with weakness or shortness of breath, nerve damage with weakness in limbs, pregnancy complications, mental confusion, forgetfulness or other cognitive declines, mental depression, sore or swollen tongue, peptic or mouth ulcers, headaches, heart palpitations, irritability, behavioral disorders, homocysteine accumulation, DNA synthesis and repair are impaired and this could lead to cancer development. Large uptake in patients with ischaemic heart disease may also lead to increased rates of cancer.[8]

H. **VITAMIN B12:** Cobalamin has a cobalt atom in it hence our need for cobalt as a trace mineral and the danger of radioactive fallout which has a high concentration of a radioactive isotope of cobalt. This gets in to B12 in nature and then that is how it gets into our bodies. There are a bunch of these including:

* Cyanocobalamin – Not found in nature.
* Hydroxocobalamin
* Methylcobalamin – An active NATURAL form of Vitamin B12.
* Adenosylcobalamin – Another active form of Vitamin B12. The Cyano- form is manufactured and often found in supplements. Personally I would prefer a naturally occurring form. Who, (and I mean, which greedy monster billionaire) determined that the cheaply made cyanocobalamin is exactly the same as the naturally occurring forms, so just dump it down the people's throats, who cares? Methylcobalamin has been used: in sleep-wake rhythm disorders, to protect the cognitive function of patients suffering chronic fatigue syndrome, stroke, depression, Alzheimer's disease and other neurological disorders. It is believed that methylcobalamin may help to remove brain-damaging levels of the neurotransmitter glutamate. Trials have reported that it reduces neurotoxicity and lowers excess glutamate levels. This in turn promotes the reduction of fatigue, stabilization of mood, improvement of memory and executive brain function.[9]

I digress here a bit to mention another B vitamin, B17, known as Amygdalin or neoamygdalin and erroneously as laetrile. The latter is manufactured and is not the same compound and should never be taken under any circumstances. The naturally occurring amygdalin or neoamygdalin are not essential nutrients, and therefore they should not be referred to as a "Vitamin" for the human body and are found in bitter almonds and apricot pits. It is believed that they decompose into D-glucose, benzaldehyde, and prussic acid (a.k.a cyanide, a DEADLY POISON) but this happens in the presence of SULFURIC acid and in hydrochloric acid, the one found in HUMAN STOMACHS, it decomposes into mandelic acid, D-glucose, and ammonia; granted also not the loveliest, but at least you won't die from cyanide poisoning.

Laetrile was marketed as a cancer cure and there are plenty who believe that the FDA, the AMA, and the big pharmaceuticals are hiding the fact that it works. I have my serious doubts and do not recommend laetrile because it is an artificial compound, does not occur in nature, and is not one of the naturally occurring forms. I also do not advocate any form of "Vitamin" B17 for any reason either because the FDA and the AMA might be right about their toxicity and the fact is they will put me in jail if I say otherwise.

I also digress here a little more since I have already given you a massive amount of information. One important caution: just because you have many of the symptoms listed under a particular nutrient's deficiency, does not mean that is what is wrong with you. This is important enough that I will say it again, in bold: **WARNING: NEVER DIAGNOSE YOURSELF, UNLESS YOU ARE A LICENSED, PRACTICING MEDICAL DOCTOR.** If you are suffering from serious symptoms such as any that are listed above, then, even if you are suffering from a vitamin deficiency, you should still take yourself to a doctor immediately. There are plenty of cases in which a person suffers from the deficiency, not because it is lacking in their diet, but because their body has a much more complicated problem where it fails to absorb or utilize the nutrient even when it is present in sufficient quantities. Short version: get yourself to a doctor and get the proper diagnosis if you are suffering from any kinds of serious symptoms.

I. **CHOLINE:** This is a macronutrient closely related to the other vitamin B molecules and is sometimes called Vitamin B4, but this is not universally accepted. It is present in animal fat tissue but it happens to be water soluble making it, like all of the other B vitamins, relatively safe to consume in excess. Choline plays a vital role in the creation of DNA during cell division but it plays many other roles throughout the human body just like the rest of the B complex. Choline deficiency is rare and usually related to digestive and liver illness (failure of digestive system to be able to absorb it from the foods we eat.) Deficiency is nasty and similar to many B vitamin deficiency diseases and includes the following symptoms: fatigue, memory loss, cognitive decline, learning disabilities, muscle aches and nerve damage. [10] Typical of the B vitamins you could experience any one, some, or all of these symptoms and still not be sure which B vitamin is causing the trouble. IF YOU EXPERIENCE ANY SERIOUS SYMPTOMS FOR OVER ONE DAY. THEN YOU SHOULD SEE A DOCTOR.

THE VITAMIN B COMPLEX

All of the B vitamins contribute to two main kinds of processes in the human body: 1) Proper BRAIN and NERVOUS SYSTEM function, and 2) Cell division and proper maintenance of the DNA in all cells in the body. While not many people are dying of beriberi and pellagra these days, chronic deficiency means that day after day for weeks even months, the person is not getting even the conservative RDA amounts and that can and will MESS WITH YOUR BRAIN and therefore your MIND. And the effects occur so subtly that you will not even notice that it is happening, but it can and will make you miserable in many different ways. Chronic deficiency will also lead to stress on all cell division throughout the body which slows organ regeneration which is always taking place and it can set you up for cancer (corrupted DNA in any single cell can start that process.) So be sure to get your B's.

3. **VITAMIN C:** a.k.a. Ascorbic acid. Well, there is a lot of research into this one. Suffice it to say that without it, you get brown spots on the skin, spongy gums, bleeding gums, tooth loss lethargy, and death from the disease known as Scurvy. There are a lot of reports that this vitamin doesn't help prevent occurrences of the common cold, to reports that it does prevent a wide variety of diseases including cancer itself. There is plenty of debate about what the RDA should be with the government vacillating with numbers in the range of 45mg to 95mg per day while most humans inadvertently consume many times this amount anyway.[11] Since it is difficult to overdose on Vitamin C (but it is possible) I would recommend staying below 3000mg and I would recommend taking ONLY NATURALLY EXTRACTED forms containing specifically L-Ascorbic acid ONLY.

4. **VITAMIN D:** Another well studied vitamin with no less than five variants. The only one of interest to us however should be Vitamin D3 which is the one you make in your skin when exposed to sunlight. It probably takes about 20 minutes for this process to be effective and sunblock will not help you here because it is the ultraviolet radiation, which the sunblock really blocks, that is the one that powers the Vitamin D synthesis. I would recommend getting at least two 20 minute exposures to full sunlight per day, and this means at least the face and the arms. In lieu of this a natural extract of Vitamin D3 can be taken. Deficiency results in malformed and weakened bones in particular, and supplementation is recommended, along with calcium, in order to avoid many bone ailments including the very common malady osteoporosis which I should point out,

should not be nearly as common as it is and I suspect that this is due to either the chronic POISONING of our bodies due to the POISONS in our food, or it is due to nuclear fallout or chemical contaminants in the environment like DDT or another of my favorites, fluorinated water (more on this miserable POISON in a later volume.) Vitamin D is readily made in the body by the liver, the skin and the kidneys, the intermediate form created by the kidneys is used by certain cells in the immune system to create a form that attacks invading organisms (like bacteria.) The form made by the skin is the one that promotes healthy coordination of the growth of the bones.[12]

5. **VITAMIN E:** a.k.a. x-Tocopherol and the Tocotrienols. This family of compounds has many cellular metabolic functions, but the most important function of note is that this is an oil soluble ANTIOXIDANT. There are studies that suggest that excesses are toxic which I would believe based on the fact that this is not a water soluble nutrient, and those tend to be dangerous. On the other hand there are studies involving megadosages with no noticeable toxicity reports.[13] Being an oil soluble I would err on the side of caution and keep this one at no more than 2 to 3 times the RDA.

    A. α-tocopherol: (alpha) is the most biologically active and the second most commonly found in the North American diet. Being a fat soluble ANTIOXIDANT makes Vitamin E one of the more valuable nutrients in the direct removal of TOXINS that CAUSE CANCER.

    B. γ-tocopherol: (gamma) is the most common form.

6. **VITAMIN K:** a family of compounds first discovered to assist in the coagulation of the blood. Vitamin K has been linked to proper utilization of insulin and therefore proper blood sugar regulation as well as heart health and even helps prevent cancer. The NATURALLY OCCURING K1 and K2 have shown NO SIGNS OF TOXICITY in studies so far.[14]

    A. K1: a.k.a. phylloquinone, this is the variant that most plants create and likely an OK one for you in reasonable amounts (no more than 2 to 5 times the RDA.)

    B. K2: a.k.a. menaquinone, this one is synthesized by bacteria in the small intestine (they convert K1 into K2), and is likely the one we mostly rely on and is non-toxic and possibly a requirement as well as K1.

    C. K3, K4, K5: ALL MANUFACTURED and have shown evidence in studies that they are TOXIC and should be avoided.

    This last point is critical. ALL MANUFACTURED forms of Vitamin K have been studied and in clinical trials have shown evidence that they are toxic. If you don't believe me you can go on a month long odyssey on the Internet like I did to find the reports and then find that they mysteriously vanish the next day. But my point is, if it hasn't already sunk in: what our sorcerers cook up in their pots is not the same as what the plants produce after millions of years of coevolution – and that's the key, co-evolution. We and the plants and animals all evolved together over millions of years and now some punk comes along who can do a little math and in a month is going to simmer up some crap in a test tube and tell me that its not only good for me but that its BETTER for me than eggs, milk, red meat, etc, that all co-evolved with humans over millions of years? And that is a flat out LIE.

Let me ask you this: if all that nature provides is so bad, and evil, and toxic, then how did mankind survive at all? Answer: because nothing found in nature is bad for you except snakes, wasps, tigers, poison ivy and angry elephants. In other words, we know that certain species have developed poisons as their methods of defense and there are no mysteries as to which ones they are; the rest are things we and our predecessors have been happily and healthily consuming for millions of years.

Many argue that we weren't healthy as a species and I contend that this is another total LIE. If, as a species we had not been healthy, then not only would we not have survived, we would not have kept EVOLVING UPWARDS to have bigger and more powerful BRAINS. That big fat brain in our heads is not just an incomprehensibly complex evolutionary achievement, it is also a very demanding and delicate organ. A chronic shortage of any nutrient especially as a fetus, newborn, or in early childhood will result in dramatically reduced brain function. So I refuse to believe that the average proto-human up through the eons was a skin and bones half-starved malnourished wretch dropping dead in his teens. If this were the case, that brain would have never developed much less persisted and IMPROVED through all of those eons.

Here's another interesting tidbit you should think about: did you know that oceanic lobsters have some hormones that are identical to those found in the human body and that they perform the same functions? What's the point? The point is that these creatures' ancestors appeared in the oceans at least 400,000,000 years ago; long before we appeared on the planet and yet they have some chemistry that is identical to ours. Why? Because we are RELATED to them. Rather distantly to be sure, but we, like all life forms on Earth, are related to all other life forms on the planet and when the lobsters developed a successful piece of biochemistry, it was passed on to the subsequent evolutionary offspring who didn't bother changing it, since it already worked.

When early proto-humans evolved, they evolved made out of the same stuff, the exact same genetic material, cellular construction, and chemistry as EVERYTHING else around them; plant and animal. So which came first, the apple trees and the cows, or humans? The apples trees and the cows were here first and we evolved later but made out of the same stuff and only because we are made out of the same stuff as everything else were we able to snap an apple off of those trees and gobble it down and occasionally get lucky enough to spear a cow and cut it up and barbeque it for dinner and there cannot be a cobbled-up concoction in a test tube made with the accumulated knowledge of mankind over the last few hundred years that could possibly replace the food we are supposed to eat that is made out of the stuff we are made out of and that possesses trillions of atoms and molecules in forms that we may never fully understand or be able to exactly duplicate.

And why should we want to cobble up a grape in a test tube anyway other than the scientific challenge of actually achieving it when all you have to do if you want a grape is just plant the seed, water it, and wait for it to flower and fruit. No gigantic facility, complicated instruments, and rooms full of stuck-up self-aggrandizing jackasses required; just seed, dirt, water, sun, patience = bowl full of grapes. Done.

That concludes the rant and the list of regular Vitamins as they have been named as such. It is important to note that there are plenty of nutrients that the body needs, that are not called vitamins but it makes them no less important to consider. There are also many important and active natural substances that are NOT needed on a regular basis by the body and these would properly be referred to as, at best, supplements, but I prefer to call them REMEDIALS, things that can shore up some problem, or even treat some chronic ailment, but unless the need exists, they should most often be kept to a minimum if taken at all.

One of the most significant sets of NUTRIENTS (I use the word to mean ESSENTIAL, and without which you would get sick and even die) are the minerals. I'll go over these in the next book but it is important to note the FORM, in the case of the minerals. For example, we all know that iron is an important mineral, but in what form? You are certainly not going to go around licking pure iron nails … or even grinding up rust (iron oxides) in your tea. Yet, many multivitamins include the metallic minerals as oxides which is basically how most of these are found in the Earth's crust, so they are basically selling you rocks to eat. Thanks, but not only is this as unappetizing as it sounds, it is also as useless to your body and your ability to absorb it as it would be to sit down and begin gnawing on a rock.

There is a good reason why we gnaw on carrots and apples rather than rocks; because we cannot digest rocks and we cannot extract any nutrients from them; that's what the carrot plants and the apple trees do for a living and why we are supposed to gnaw on the fruits of their labor and not rocks. That's why they taste good and rocks taste, well, like rocks.

END OF CHAPTER QUIZ

1. Which is the B vitamins should be taken carefully and in moderation?
   A. Thiamine
   B. Niacin
   C. Riboflavin
   D. Biotin

ANSWER: B. Niacin. Although it would take a massive quantity of any B vitamin to present serious side effects, Niacin can cause a reaction in amounts as small as double or triple the RDA amount.

2. Which form of Vitamin A is dangerous (to take in large quantities)?
   A. Retinol
   B. Beta-carotene
   C. All forms
   D. No form is dangerous in large quantities

Answer: A. Retinol. Beta-carotene is a very safe antioxidant form and the reason carrots are orange. Many fruits and vegetables ranging in color from red to orange to yellow are so because of the beta-carotene and it is very good for you even in moderate excess.

3. alpha-Tocopherol is the naturally occurring form of:
   A. Vitamin A
   B. Vitamin K
   C. Vitamin D
   D. Vitamin E

Answer: D. Vitamin E

1. Which Vitamin in extreme excess could lead to excessive blood clotting possibly causing heart attack or stroke?
   A. Vitamin A
   B. Vitamin K
   C. Vitamin D
   D. Vitamin E

Answer: B. Vitamin K. Although natural forms (K1 and K2) are considered far less dangerous than the manufactured forms.

2. Which Vitamin promotes healthy skin and bones?
   A. Vitamin A
   B. Vitamin K
   C. Vitamin D
   D. Vitamin E

Answer: C. Vitamin D

3. Which Vitamin cannot be synthesized by the human body (and must be in our food in order to get it)?
   A. Vitamin B3
   B. Vitamin B12
   C. Vitamin C
   D. Vitamin D

Answer: Vitamin C

CHAPTER 4 – NATURAL SOURCES OF THE VITAMINS

Before anyone goes running break-neck to the pharmacy, they should ALWAYS consider getting their essential nutrients from natural sources FIRST.

If mankind was healthy enough as a hunter-gatherer a million years ago to be able to evolve into the high mental capacity species he is now; then nature does indeed provide us with everything we need. Only in those special cases in which the person has little access to an abundance of fresh foods would they BE FORCED to rely on pills to get the nutrients they need.

VITAMIN A

While true Vitamin A (retinol and retinal) are almost exclusively found only in animal products like eggs, beta-carotene is a compound found in abundance in raw edible plant foods. Beta-carotene is not exactly Vitamin A, but the liver can convert it into "true" Vitamin A on demand and beta-carotene is water-soluble, non-toxic and the body can store it for later use. It does store it in the skin and I have met someone who turned ORANGE (literally!) from eating too many carrots. Even at that level it is still non-toxic though I personally don't want to turn bright orange.

While some plants actually have higher levels of beta-carotene than carrots, the good news is that carrots are easily found in most grocery stores and open market places. And the best news of all: just ONE medium sized raw carrot contains about 200% of the RDA listed amount of Vitamin A albeit in the form of beta-carotene that does have to be processed by the liver in order to become usable as Vitamin A.[1]

I personally eat at least one a day and usually plenty more than that and I haven't turned orange either.

TOP NATURAL SOURCE OF VITAMIN A:

FOOD	AMT(%RDA)
WINTER/BUTTERNUT SQUASH (1 cup)	450%
SWEET POTATO (1 medium, cooked)	450%
BEEF LIVER (1oz.)	178%
CARROT (1 medium, raw)	200%

(Beef liver is the highest content superfood source of true Vitamin A in the form of Retinol. The plant sources are all in the form of beta-carotene.)[1]

VITAMIN B1 – THIAMINE

Vitamin B1 is critical to the human body and prolonged deficiency can lead to many nasty symptoms and ultimately death. The good news is that it is found in most natural foods to some degree, but I prefer to know that I have my bases covered.

TOP SOURCES OF THIAMINE:

FOOD	AMT(%RDA)
1 Cup SUNFLOWER SEEDS	164%
1 Cup GREEN PEAS (cooked)	40%

Herring and salmon are good sources as well.[2]
VITAMIN B2 – RIBOFLAVIN
This is another critical B vitamin that is also found in most natural foods. It does turn out to be difficult to find it in EFFECTIVE (complete 100% RDA) QUANTITIES in any particular food source, however, and since it is a fundamental daily requirement that is a PROBLEM.

Based on the fact that it is not particularly abundant in most specific food sources means that most people are probably not getting enough riboflavin in their regular diet unless they are eating vitamin fortified foods like some breakfast cereals. But those breakfast cereals are based on LOW QUALITY PROCESSED GRAIN MASS which is at best a SECONDARY FOOD SOURCE and not the best thing to be eating on a daily basis.

Although riboflavin is found in just about all foods from plant to animal matter, it is not there in sufficient quantities to add up over the course of the day to an acceptable amount and if there is ONE VITAMIN that you NEED that you are probably not getting enough of, it is riboflavin. For this vitamin alone, it is very much worth it to seek out a high quality B complex vitamin pill and take it daily if you can't get 100% RDA daily from your regular daily diet of natural whole foods.

TOP SOURCES OF RIBOFLAVIN:

FOOD	AMT(%RDA)
Beef liver (3 oz.)	>100%
Lamb (3 oz.)	>100%
Milk (1 cup)	26%
Egg (1 large)	13%

I personally ABHOR beef liver and I don't get very many opportunities to buy lamb meat and I am not going to chug down a quart of milk or eat 8 eggs a day. So I hope from this you can see that we do NEED to take at the very least a Vitamin B2 (Riboflavin) supplement or eat plenty of beef liver and/or lamb.[3]
VITAMIN B3 – NIACIN
This is a well known and well studied B vitamin going back almost a century. Niacin deficiency leads to the malady known as pellagra which was common in the 1700's in the U.S. because corn became the main staple of the colonial diet. Anyone who eats mainly processed foods made from corn and wheat flour (low nutritional value foods) is susceptible to Niacin deficiency issues and the disease is still prevalent in poor and undeveloped regions worldwide. Fortunately; there are foods that are rich in niacin and it is a safe vitamin to take in excess and I make sure I get plenty in my daily natural whole foods diet.

TOP SOURCES OF NIACIN:

FOOD	AMT.
Turkey or chicken (6 oz. white meat)	≈100%
Peanuts (1/2 cup)	≈100%

Tuna (6 oz.)   ≈100%
Beef (9 oz. organic – grass-fed)   ≈100%

I have no problem sitting down to a nice thick 9 oz. steak, but not every single day! And niacin is not absent from poultry dark meat, just in lower concentrations. Since ALL of the B vitamins, are involved in complex biochemical processes throughout the human body and deficiencies lead to low energy and mess with your brain chemistry causing mood problems as well as far more sinister trouble like lack of concentration and ultimately dementia, it is a VERY GOOD IDEA to make sure you are getting a healthy dose in your daily diet to stay not only healthy but also in a FUNCTIONAL STATE OF MIND as well.[4]

VITAMIN B5 – PANTOTHENIC ACID

"Pantos" is Greek for "everywhere." And pantothenic acid is indeed found in most foods, however, just like riboflavin (B2) it is probably not enough to satisfy our THRIVE-LEVEL daily requirements. Pantothenic acid deficiency disease is very rare because it is found in most foods, but prolonged periods of insufficient intake of the vitamin can and will have consequences. You might not die from this but it will – just like all of the other B vitamins – affect your metabolism (make you physically weak and tired) and your mood (feelings of depression and confusion.) Pantothenic acid is the other B vitamin that I believe most people are not getting in sufficient quantities to live at OPTIMUM HEALTH and you should consider making certain that you are getting enough in your natural whole foods daily diet or if absolutely necessary by taking a GOOD daily B complex supplement in order to shore up this vitamin whose deficiency is EPIDEMIC in our society.

TOP SOURCES OF PANTOTHENIC ACID:

FOOD   AMT.
Chicken liver (4 oz. organic)   >100%
Sunflower seeds (5 oz.)   100%

You will never find me waiting in line for chicken liver! Animal livers are not on my "top food choices" list because they – just like our own liver – filter out POISONS from what the animals are eating and are potentially LOADED with those poisons. And it is difficult at best to investigate the farms that are the sources of the animals that we are buying in the grocery stores to make sure that they are in a clean environment and being fed healthy food and being treated properly. All of these factors would combine to mean "organic" to me, but the FDA is allowing this label on many foods that do not necessarily meet my criteria and they probably wouldn't meet your criteria either.

I do consume a LOT of sunflower seed kernels daily (they are a SUPERFOOD if ever there was such a thing) but I still take my GOOD B complex on those occasions when I can't because I am busy or traveling just to be sure I get enough B5.[5]

VITAMIN B6 – PYRIDOXINE
This vitamin is used to synthesize Vitamin B3 in the body, it also plays over ONE HUNDRED other known cellular functions including the formation of many amino acids as well as the formation of hemoglobin molecules in the blood. Suffice it to say that you better make sure you are getting plenty of Vitamin B6. B6 like many other B vitamins is present in most foods but likely not enough to provide us with THRIVE-LEVEL amounts on a daily basis.

TOP SOURCES OF VITAMIN B6 - PYRIDOXINE:

FOOD	AMT.
Turkey breast (6 oz. organic)	>100%
Pistachios (3/4 cup)	>100%
Tuna (10 oz.)	100%

That is a lot of tuna, I don't plan to eat 10 ounces every day, or that much pistachio nuts either. However, I do eat plenty of turkey and can mix in the others on the days that I don't. The very best plan to make sure that you are getting the OPTIMAL amount for THRIVE-LEVEL health if you aren't sure you are getting it on a daily basis from a natural whole foods diet is to get it from a GOOD QUALITY B complex supplement.[6]

VITAMIN B7 – BIOTIN
Biotin is critical – like all of the B vitamins – and is found in abundance in many foods. It also happens that we actually need very little, but we do need it on a daily basis because the body will rid itself of any perceived excess through the urine. Biotin deficiency is seen on occasion and is usually traced to digestive disease, heavy smoking or eating large amounts of raw egg whites on a regular basis. Raw egg whites contain a substance called avidin which binds to biotin and many other B vitamins and prevents their absorption in the digestive tract – STAY AWAY from raw or "runny" egg whites and MAYONNAISE which is made from raw eggs: they are BAD FOR YOU.

I love my eggs "over easy" but I make very certain that ALL of the egg white has been cooked and turned white. This neutralizes the avidin and makes the egg a tremendous source of… all of the B vitamins!

The average adult is said to need about 300mcg (micrograms) which is indeed a tiny amount, but pregnant and breastfeeding mothers need upwards of 35 milligrams: that's about 120 TIMES MORE than usual.

TOP SOURCES OF BIOTIN:

FOOD	AMT(mg=milligrams)
Beef liver (3 oz. organic)	27 – 35mg
Egg (1 large, properly cooked)	13 – 25mg
Salmon (3 oz.)	4 – 5mg
Cauliflower (1 cup)	0.2 – 2mg
Whole grain Bread (1 slice)	0.2 – 6mg

It is important to remember that you need Vitamin B7 on a daily basis just like ALL of the B vitamins and I try to eat at least one of the above on a daily basis so I make sure I get it. Otherwise you will have to get it in a GOOD B COMPLEX. Pregnant and breastfeeding mothers should DEFINITELY take a QUALITY biotin supplement.[7]

VITAMIN B9 – FOLIC ACID (or FOLATE)

Folic acid or folate is essential to the creation of new cells due to its role in copying and the synthesis of new DNA molecules during cell division. Since almost all organs in the human body continuously renew their tissues, a lack of folic acid would result in catastrophic weakening of all bodily systems and organs. Acute deficiency leads to anemia (improperly formed red blood cells) diminished immune system and poor digestion. People at high risk include pregnant and breastfeeding mothers, people with liver disease (that means alcoholics as well, I'm not being judgmental here, I used to be a daily guzzler myself and haven't touched that POISON in 30 years,) people on kidney dialysis, people taking medication for diabetes, as well as other diuretic medications. Clearly then kidney troubles and liver troubles can lead to shortages in the body of Folic acid.

TOP SOURCES OF B9 – FOLIC ACID or FOLATE:

FOOD	AMT.
Wheat germ (2.3 oz.)	≈100%
Chick peas (Garbanzos; (1 cup)	>100%
Beef liver (6 oz. organic)	>100%
Lentils (1 cup)	≈90%

None of these are on most folk's daily diet and most of the rest of the natural foods that we eat have much lower quantities. As such it is very likely that most people are getting SOME Folic acid but not enough to meet our THRIVE-LEVEL requirements, especially those folks in the at-risk list above. I now eat Wheat germ in my oatmeal at least four times a week. Be sure to take a GOOD B Complex that includes ample Folic acid if you are not eating these Folate rich sources daily.[8]

VITAMIN B12 – METHYLCOBALAMIN

This is the BIG ONE: some experts estimate that up to 10% of all Americans are B12 deficient and that is STAGGERING and one of the main reasons I insist that the "First World" nations including Europe and much of Asia are the BEST FED and MOST MALNOURISHED societies the world have ever seen. Oh, we shovel down food by the pound, but it is mostly SECONDARY foods like grains and starchy roots (like potatoes) and BEANS all of which MUST BE COOKED in order to become EDIBLE.

What's worse is that THIS vitamin is only found in TRACE quantities if it is found at all in any plant. This is THE animal vitamin so vegetarians and strict vegans NEED to be aware of this shortcoming and find a way to get B12. In fact, I would guess that the reason B12 deficiency is so prevalent in the U.S. is precisely because vegetarianism is so prevalent in this country.

Like ALL B vitamins, B12 deficiency is nasty business and it will result in the degradation of all organ systems because it plays a role in the formation of DNA and deficiency results in anemia as well as terrible effects on the human brain including depression, anxiety and confusion.

Ever wonder why so many vegetarians are pale as a white bed sheet and have a glassy eyed stare? That is CLASSIC VITAMIN B12 DEFICIENCY SYNDROME. I have no quarrels with the vegetarians; I am 90% vegetarian myself, BUT if you are going to pursue that lifestyle – and it is a lifestyle choice and has NOTHING TO DO with our "natural diet" as humans (you have CANINES in your mouth for a REASON: they are CARNIVORE teeth. We have carnivorous equipment because we evolved eating meat) then you MUST find a way to supplement your diet with Vitamin B12. Prolonged and chronic Vitamin B12 deficiency will lead to systemic degradation of all systems in the human body and such a person will be sickly and suffer from reduced mental function. Vegan's who refuse to even take any product derived from animals are at an especially high risk of Vitamin B12 issues especially as they get older. The aging body is one that is gradually breaking down anyway – even if it is getting everything at the THRIVE-LEVEL, but after decades of chronic B12 deficiency these people are at very high risk of just about anything and everything going wrong from catastrophic immune failure (dying during a short stay at the hospital due to a pneumonia infection, for example) to dementia/Alzheimer's disease.

That should be ample warning that we all need to make very sure that we are getting a THRIVE-LEVEL supply of Vitamin B12 on a daily basis. As for the vegetarians, I am on their side, I want to help them achieve their goal of remaining vegetarians if that is what they want. But it is critical to point out that virtually ALL supplements on the shelves of the big stores and pharmacies contain CYANOCOBALAMIN which is SYNTHETIC and it is NOT the molecule found in animal products or our own bodies which is METHYLCOBALAMIN. I don't know which greedy money-grubbing billionaire slimeball paid which laboratory to proclaim that the two are the same but they are NOT.

There are many GOOD products that can be found on the Internet that have the CORRECT and NATURAL form of B12 – methylcobalamin – in them and unfortunately for the vegans, they are extracted from animal sources. I would highly recommend that in this ONE CASE, that the vegans make an exception and refuse to take the ARTIFICIAL and potentially DEADLY synthetic version and take the natural one instead. I know I refuse to take that manmade garbage just like I refuse to eat anything with that infernal Yellow DEADLY, PROVEN CARCINOGEN, number five in it and for the same reason: if some punk cooked it up then it is thousands of times more likely to KILL than to HELP.

TOP SOURCES OF VITAMIN B12 – METHYLCOBALAMIN:

FOOD	AMT.
Beef liver (1 oz. organic)	≈300%
Sardines (3 oz.)	>100%
Atlantic mackerel (3 oz.)	>100%

After these sources the amounts fall off sharply and usually require you to eat far too much of the food to be practical: an egg has 11% of the daily requirement. I don't know about you but I am not about to eat 9 eggs a day. And sardines or mackerel are not at the top of my daily diet list either and you already know my opinion of beef liver aside from the fact that it is pasty and not so tasty (to me, if you like it then go for it, it is one of the top SUPERFOODS, just make sure those cows live in a clean, free environment and are not subjected to exposure to chemicals like pesticides in particular.)

You can bet I order my vitamins online and get a GOOD B complex that includes METHYLCOBALAMIN from natural animal sources: THAT is exactly what separates the GOOD B vitamin supplements from the BAD ONES.[9]

CHOLINE – THE "SORT OF" B VITAMIN

Like most of the B vitamins to which this compound is related, choline plays a critical role in upwards of a hundred different cellular functions throughout the body and is known to play a critical role in proper brain and nerve function. Deficiency disease is rare and the symptoms are similar to the rest of the B vitamins including fatigue and reduced mental capacity and it is therefore very much worth while to make sure you are getting enough choline on a daily basis.

There are no major "superfoods" containing ample amounts of choline, but we do manufacture some for ourselves. Nevertheless, because we know that the RDA's can be rather low, you should strive to make sure you get at least 100% of the daily requirement if not plenty more and that might have to include a supplement to be absolutely certain you are getting enough of this essential nutrient.

TOP SOURCES OF CHOLINE:

FOOD	AMT.
Beef liver (3 oz. organic)	≈50%
Salmon (1 fillet)	≈50%
Egg (1 large)	≈27%

So a breakfast of two to three eggs will get you over half way there and 3 ounces of beef liver or a salmon fillet (unfortunately my source did not say the weight, and salmon can be very large fish!) will finish the job. I will discuss how I manage to get liver into my diet in a later chapter.[10]

VITAMIN C – L-ASCORBIC ACID

This is one of the first vitamins ever identified and it is one of the most thoroughly studied on them all. Yet, most products on the shelves of the stores contain artificial ascorbic acid. The problem with this is that the molecule happens to be a stereoenantiomer. Now that's fancy chemist-speak for any molecule that has a 3-dimensional structure that would allow for at least two different versions based on the 3-dimensional arrangement of their atoms allowing for so-called "left-handed" versions as well as "right-handed" versions which would otherwise be identical. You have heard of "left-handed" sugar which tastes like normal sugar but does not get absorbed by the human body and thus yields zero calories. Likewise, when they make Vitamin C, it yields 50% right-handed ascorbic acid and 50% of the left-handed form.

And there is mounting evidence that the "wrong-way" or artificial form comprising 50% of the synthetic Vitamin C is actually TOXIC to our bodies. Taking the artificial version of Vitamin C is sort of like telling an alcoholic to take his liver medication dissolved in a martini: self-defeating and ridiculous.

Living things have been around for a very long time, the green plants can trace their heritage back over a billion years to the earliest forms of life on Earth including the cyanobacteria – the first organisms on Earth that used photosynthesis to create sugar for their energy. The green plants over time have optimized themselves and ALL plants make ONLY the right-handed sugar molecules and they also ALL ONLY make the correct version of Vitamin C which is L-ascorbic acid. Then we came along and we evolved taking in ONLY this version of the molecule and this is the only one we need and the ONLY one we should be taking into our bodies as well.

It is incredibly difficult to find a supplement that is made from pure natural sources and thus ONLY HAS the correct L-ascorbic acid in it and NONE of the "wrong-way" manmade version in it.

The good news is that many plants and fruits in particular are LOADED with Vitamin C and these are highly preferred if you cannot find a supplement made from pure natural sources that ONLY HAS the L-ascorbic acid in it.

TOP SOURCES OF VITAMIN C – L-ASCORBIC ACID:

FOOD	AMT.
Acerola berry (1 small berry)	≈100%
Kiwi (2 fruits)	≈100%
Guava (1 average sized fruit)	≈200%
Orange (1 average sized)	≈100%
Grapefruit (1 average sized)	≈100%

No doubt the vegetarians are rejoicing about the quantity and quality of the Vitamin C they are getting in their daily diet. And they are quite correct, the fruits are the best source of Vitamin C on Earth and we DO NOT MAKE IT in our bodies and chronic deficiency will result in bleeding gums, tooth loss, depressed immune system (even though some of the "experts" insist that there is no definitive clinical evidence of this) and eventual death if the amounts stay too low. But remember that the RDA of 45mg to 95mg is a very conservative estimate and the amount was originally set as that amount necessary to avoid getting scurvy (the name of the disease that kills you due to chronic deficiency of Vitamin C) and has nothing to do with the amount needed for OPTIMAL HEALTH; the THRIVE-LEVEL amount hat we want to take on a daily basis. I do take the L-ascorbic acid supplement, but I also eat citrus on a daily basis as well so I know I am getting plenty of Vitamin C and even though smoking depletes Vitamin C (yes, I admit I am a heavy smoker, no one's perfect) I haven't had a cold or flu as far back as I can remember.[11]

VITAMIN D - CHOLECALCIFEROL

Just about everybody knows that Vitamin D is necessary for the formation of strong bones and teeth. But it has many more roles than that in the human body including proper immune response and brain function.

Vitamin D is also fairly uncommon in our natural foods and this is exactly why we can manufacture it ourselves in the skin.

Vitamin D deficiency is far more common in the industrialized nations than most people think and this is because most people are not drinking a quart of milk every day (I certainly do not want to do that) and they are not getting enough sun (I certainly do not want to get deep fried by overexposure to short wave ultraviolet radiation either.) I recommend however, that you do make the effort to get your Vitamin D from natural sources including at least two 20 minute exposures to the sun each day. I work in my garden daily so I know I get sufficient exposure to the sun (face and arms is all that is required) and one of my many coffee's that I drink each day is a café con leche so I at least get one cup of straight up milk (plus that infernal coffee of course) each day as well. If you are going to depend on a supplement (which I also take occasionally) be sure that it is NOT AN ARTIFICIAL FORM.

TOP SOURCES OF VITAMIN D:

SOURCE	AMT.
Sunlight (total 40 minutes face and arms)	≈100%
Cod liver oil (1 teaspoon)	≈150%
Salmon (3 oz. wild-caught)	≈100%
Tuna (8 oz.)	≈100%
Milk (1 cup, fortified)	≈31%

So it isn't the milk that is getting me enough Vitamin D, it is the sunlight. If you do not want to drink a quart of fortified milk each day or get out in the sun, then I recommend that tablespoon of Cod Liver Oil; it is real natural Vitamin D3.[12]

VITAMIN E – alpha-TOCOPHEROL

Vitamin E is found in many foods and deficiency disease is rare and usually associated with digestive troubles that prevent the absorption of fats. Vitamin E is a fat soluble vitamin like Vitamin A but it is not nearly as dangerous as Vitamin A in excess but extreme excesses should be avoided nonetheless.

Vitamin E is a powerful antioxidant and plays a key role in our immune health, skin health, vision, and prevents genetic mutation (assists in gene replication during cellular division) and may be a key to cancer prevention (that is a personal opinion, but the implication is rather obvious.)

TOP SOURCES OF VITAMIN E:

FOOD	AMT.
Wheat germ (1/2 cup)	≈100%
Sunflower seeds (1/2 cup)	≈100%
Almonds (3 oz.)	≈100%

Vitamin E is found in most nuts, but almonds have the most by a large margin. In other words, because nuts are so high in fat (even though it is the good, polyunsaturated kind) you would have to eat a large quantity of them to get your daily requirement and they can make you gain weight.

You might have noticed that sunflower seeds are turning up quite often. I eat unsalted sunflower kernels DAILY – they are one of nature's true SUPERFOODS. Because of Vitamin E's antioxidant properties and the fact that it assists the proper coordination of the genes during cell division I HIGHLY RECOMMEND that you make sure that you are getting a good dose of natural Vitamin E on a daily basis: somewhere between 100% and 250% at most, but do not exceed that! Remember, this is an OIL SOLUBLE vitamin and NOT a water soluble vitamin like most of the others so it is possible to overdose on Vitamin E because your body cannot get rid of it easily like the water soluble nutrients.[13]

VITAMIN K – PHYLLOQUINONE or MENAQUINONE

Vitamin K has been much maligned because it "causes blood clots." This however could only happen in cases of extreme overindulgence. While Vitamin K does indeed help the blood to clot when this is necessary due to injury, Vitamin E happens to prevent internal blood clots from happening. So if you are taking sufficient quantities of ALL vitamins, minerals and other essential nutrients, then Vitamin K will not harm you in moderate excess at all and it is, like all essential nutrients involved in so many different biochemical processes within the human body that we might NEVER figure them all out.

Vitamin K has been linked to proper utilization of insulin in the human body and chronic Vitamin K deficiency could lead to blood sugar issues like hypoglycemia and possibly even diabetes. This is exactly why doctors always tell diabetics to eat more green leafy vegetables which are loaded with Vitamin K.

Vitamin K deficiency leads to easy bruising, excessive bleeding, tooth decay and weakening of the bones and I strongly suspect chronic deficiency is one of the causes of the prevalence of osteoporosis and brittle bones in the elderly. If you decide to increase your intake of Vitamin K you should also increase your intake of Vitamin E too which prevents internal blood clotting just to be on the safe side and I HIGHLY ENCOURAGE YOU TO DO SO.

TOP SOURCES OF VITAMIN K:

FOOD	AMT.
Spinach (1/2 cup)	≈500%
Cabbage (1/2 cup)	≈100%
Brussels sprouts (1/2 cup)	≈100%

Vitamin K1, a.k.a. phylloquinone, is found in the plants and K2, a.k.a. menaquinone is found in the animal products like dairy and is also manufactured by the good bacteria in our digestive tract. K3, K4, and K5 are all SYNTHETIC and are ALL suspected of being TOXIC – DO NOT TAKE THEM. Instead just add some fresh spinach leaves to your daily green tossed salad and you know you are getting plenty of Vitamin K.[14]

END OF CHAPTER QUIZ

1. Which of the following are NOT water soluble and potentially dangerous if you take too much of them?
    A. Vitamin B1 and B2
    B. Vitamin B3 and C
    C. Vitamin D and K
    D. Vitamin A and E
    Answer: D. Vitamin A and Vitamin E are both OIL soluble and you should take no more than 100% of Vitamin A on a daily basis and never in excess if you are suffering from weight problems and no more than 250% of the RDA of Vitamin E.

2. Which vitamin is not manufactured in the human body and must come from the foods we eat, and we need a LOT of it?
    A. Vitamin B3
    B. Vitamin B12
    C. Vitamin C
    D. Vitamin D
    Answer: C. Vitamin C. We can manufacture the others, but we may not make as much as we need. Only young folks in prime health that are getting plenty of exercise and eating properly and NOT indulging in junk food and processed food full of artificial additives would be likely to make all of the vitamins that they need in sufficient quantities.

3. Which vitamin is directly linked to decreased mental function such as depression and confusion?
    A. Vitamin A
    B. Vitamin B5

C. Vitamin E

D. Vitamin K

Answer: B. Vitamin B5. As a matter of fact ALL B vitamins have been linked to decreased mental function which includes everything from lack of concentration to dementia and deficiencies that severely and adversely affect the brain should be avoided because they start a "slippery slope" of decline. Once a person gets depressed and has memory loss and lack of concentration, etc. then they tend to prefer to stay that way rather than snap out of it.

4. Which food has the highest concentration of Vitamin K?

A. Sunflower seeds

B. Cod liver oil

C. Beef liver

D. Spinach

Answer: D. Spinach. Popeye had it right. I just hope he also ate plenty of sunflower seeds which are full of Vitamin E to prevent internal blood clotting!

5. The very best natural source of Vitamin D is:

A. Milk

B. Brussels sprouts

C. Sunflower seeds

D. Sunlight

Answer: D. Sunlight. A few brief exposures of about 20 minutes at a time with at least the face and arms exposed each day will allow your skin to manufacture all the Vitamin D your body needs.

6. Your best source of Vitamin A, by far is:

A. Spinach

B. Sunflower seeds

C. Beef liver

D. Carrots

Answer: D. Carrots. Even though it is in the form beta-carotene, at least ONE carrot a day will provide you with all the Vitamin A your body needs even though there are some experts who feel that you should also get animal source Vitamin A as well.

7. While Vitamin E is found in most seeds and nuts, which sources have the highest concentrations of it?

A. Sunflower seeds and Almonds

B. Peanuts and walnuts

C. Brazil nuts

D. All of the above have sufficient amounts of Vitamin E

Answer: A. Although most nuts have some Vitamin E in them, Sunflower seeds and Almonds have the highest concentration of this valuable vitamin.

Again, I am not really here to bash any particular name brand of product, and taking anything, even rocks, is better than not taking anything at all, but while you might absorb 1% of the rock dust you are taking in the form of one of the minerals in the form of its oxide, you will do much better taking the mineral in a form that you absorb MOST of what you bought. These supplements are not cheap and to pay $10 for a bottle, only to actually absorb 1% means that you will be getting 10 CENTS of what you paid for and be sending the other $9.90 cents of it right down the drain.

Remember the absorbability, solubility, and "bioactive" forms when shopping.

TIPS: Don't buy a vitamin if the company cannot be found on the Internet, and does not provide you with a land address and phone number which should be in the United States. (The government gets touchy about us buying things like this from another country.) Check the manufacturer out at the BBB and why not? If they are providing ineffective products or poisoning people with them, you ought to know right? A word on the BBB site: a company with a lot of sales will have a lot of complaints just because Americans like to whine and bellyache about every little thing and try to get everything for free – that is if they can't find a way to sue outright, which has gotten to the point that quite frankly makes me sick. But be that as it may, you want to look at percentages of customers that are upset. Small specialty companies with large numbers of complaints are to be avoided.

NATURAL SOURCE VITAMINS

Any time you can find a vendor selling vitamins extracted from natural sources, these will be the very best ones and admittedly they will be more expensive than the artificially manufactured vitamins. However, I personally would rather go without, than to consume artificially manufactured chemicals of any kind ESPECIALLY vitamins and other essential nutrients. If I am willing to PAY for these products it makes sense that I should be willing to pay for things that will make me healthy – not things that could very likely make me sick or even KILL me.

Obviously, your number one source of all of your vitamins and essential nutrients should be the food that you eat on a daily basis, but it is very difficult to find some vitamins in sufficient quantities in natural foods that we would also be willing to eat in sufficient quantities on a daily basis. For example, 3 oz. of sardines contain at least 100% of our daily requirement of Vitamin B12, and I do eat them on occasion, but I am not about to eat them daily – they are not THAT appetizing. However, if I couldn't find a supplement containing METHYLCOBALAMIN – the naturally occurring form of the vitamin – then I WOULD EAT 3 OUNCES OF SARDINES EVERY DAY. That is, natural B12 which is deeply wrapped up in brain function is a MUST; and FAKE manufactured B12 is UNACCEPTABLE. I would gladly choke down the sardines slathered in hot sauce or mustard before eating that potentially DANGEROUS manmade garbage. You have been warned.

MULTIVITAMINS

Virtually all of those "A to Z" supplements have a LOT of ingredients that are in UNUSABLE forms: this means that our digestive tracts cannot get the nutrients out of them in the forms they are putting in the pills. An excellent example of this is iron in the form of iron oxide a.k.a. RUST. We cannot digest this and only get about 1% of the iron out of the amount they are putting in the pill even though the nutrient label indicates that the pill contains 100% of the RDA of iron. This is by WEIGHT and the iron is in there in the amount they say, but our digestive tracts cannot get it out of those RUST molecules and it passes right through you and you get almost nothing from it.

And most of the rest of the ingredients are manufactured FAKE, SYNTHETIC, MANMADE versions of the nutrients. For vitamins like B12 which is KNOWN to be a different molecule from the one we need and use in our BRAINS, I am very leery of things like this. Yes, perhaps the liver can safely convert it into the one we actually use, but what if that doesn't happen in everybody? And what if that conversion process adversely affects the liver? And by adverse effect I mean KILLS liver cells in the process?

Although it is a bit more trouble to have to chase down each essential nutrient one at a time and purchase them that way and take a bowl full of pills before each meal, if they are GOOD versions of the ingredients – "biologically active" or "absorbable" or better yet, NATURAL EXTRACTS – then these are SO MUCH BETTER for you, and you GET ALL OF THE PRODUCT you are paying for, that they really are worth the extra effort.

Sometimes I coordinate which ones I am taking with my daily food regimen as well. If I plan to eat a 3 ounce can of sardines at some point during the day, then I can skip the natural source methylcobalamin B12 pill because I know I have that base covered thoroughly with the sardines.

This is a critical consideration concerning Vitamin K. If I am going to eat a ½ cup of raw spinach in my salad, then I should NOT also take my Vitamin K pill for the day. Remember that extreme excesses of Vitamin K COULD cause internal blood clotting and the best defense for that is: 1) to maintain a very healthy cardiovascular system (an upcoming "The Truth About… will cover ALL nutrients and "curative" foods that improve heart and cardiovascular health specifically,) 2) Take Vitamin E as well which prevents internal blood clotting. But because Vitamin E is an oil soluble vitamin it cannot be taken in excess either. (Only water

soluble vitamins can be easily thrown out in the urine when they
are in excess.)

So this coordination takes a little effort and a little time. I
would rather pay attention to what is going into my body and make
sure it is GOOD and SAFE and in proper amounts, than waste that
half hour watching some moronic sitcom on the boob tube. That
millionaire comedian only cares about ratings and the big fat
paycheck from the executive producers. I prefer to spend the time
making sure I OUTLIVE HIM.

PRODUCTS TO AVOID

Obviously any pills containing artificial colors, flavors or
preservatives and this would include most children's chewable
vitamins unless they specifically state that they are NOT putting
those things into the product or you read the label and don't see
them in there. (See the first chapter for the gory details on this
CANCER CAUSING GARBAGE.)

VITAMIN A

Animal sources are often recommended and there is no doubt that
they are better than beta-carotene, but most animal sources do not
contain nearly enough to satisfy our daily requirements while a
SINGLE RAW CARROT CAN fulfill our daily requirement for the
vitamin. Yes, our body does have to process the beta-carotene
into the Vitamin A for use, but it can do that and it is a completely
SAFE form of the vitamin, while straight retinol or retinal (the
animal forms) are NOT SAFE in excess. Just eat a carrot a day
and be done with it. Why spend extra money on a potentially
harmful and expensive vitamin when it is SO EASY to take care of
without all the fuss? It also solves one of my daily snacking urges
with a VERY HEALTHY, LOW CALORIE, ZERO CHOLESTEROL
snack.

CORRECT FORMS

For most vitamins you cannot go wrong if the manufacturer verifies
that they are extracted from natural sources. If this is the case then
you know you are getting the correct biologically active and
absorbable forms of the nutrients. U.S. companies rarely make this
kind of statement if it isn't true even though the FDA does not
currently regulate the sale of vitamins, minerals, and other
essential nutrients and "natural" supplements like Milk Thistle pills,
etc. However, since these OTC (Over The Counter) products are
currently a billion dollar industry, none of the major brands are
interested in LYING about their products and getting into that kind
of trouble. Nevertheless, it is always a good idea to check into
them.

Personally I don't have the time to travel to another state to
verify if the company is actually making the vitamins from natural
extract sources or if they are using manufactured chemicals, nor
do I have a fully stocked organic chemistry lab to test the products
myself. The second best thing then is to look for reviews of the

products especially by reputable reviewers like major health and wellness magazines or independent laboratories or even hospitals.
VITAMIN B1 – THIAMINE
All forms SEEM to be acceptable in any product. But I am always hesitant to buy synthetic forms even if the molecule is allegedly identical to the one that occurs in nature. Since sunflower seeds are LOADED with it and many other vitamins and minerals as well, I just buy jars of unsalted sunflower kernels and eat them straight up as one of my favorite daily snack foods and make sure I get at least ½ cup daily. The references call for a cup of sunflower seeds, not kernels which have all of the nutrients in them so a ½ cup of kernels is more than sufficient to cover your daily need of this vitamin.
VITAMIN B2 – RIBOFLAVIN
Riboflavin is found in lots of foods, but not in sufficient quantities to satisfy the 100% RDA and let's not forget that the RDA is very conservative as well. 3 oz. of beef liver or lamb will cover the requirement but they are not on my daily menu either. However, 2 cups of organic yogurt and ½ cup of spinach are on the daily menu (I cover yogurt in the next volume on Minerals and Essential Nutrients) and the spinach covers Vitamin K. Together they cover about 80% of the Riboflavin. Just ONE OUNCE of almonds contains about 20% of the RDA and will finish the job. Almonds are very high in Vitamin E as well, so in a pinch 5 oz. of almonds will give you 100% of the RDA of Vitamin B2 and E.
VITAMIN B3 – NIACIN
This is another B vitamin that I prefer to take care of in my daily eating regimen and only take the B3 pill on those occasions when I know I didn't get it during the day. I buy chicken leg quarters by the 10 pound bag and separate them out and freeze them. Usually there is anywhere from 7 to 14 of them in the bag. Either way I make sure than I am cooking over 1 pound of chicken leg quarters for dinner (either one very large one or two smaller ones) and that will knock out my niacin requirement nicely. On alternate days (no chicken or turkey burger for dinner) I can have a ½ cup of peanuts or two 5 ounce cans of tuna fish to take care of the niacin requirement. My favorite way to eat canned tuna fish is to make tuna fish salad. However, that involves one of my very favorite garnishes on Earth: mayonnaise. And this stuff is TERRIBLE FOR YOU. It is water, oil and RAW EGG WHITES blended until they become mayonnaise. And RAW EGG WHITES BIND with MOST of the B VITAMINS and prevent our digestive tract from absorbing them DEFEATING the point of eating all of that tuna fish! Now I eat the tuna fish mixed with mustard instead. Oddly, this tastes much better than you would imagine, it seems that the strong tuna flavor and the strong mustard flavor cancel each other out. Another way is to eat the tuna is with cheese either

melted cheddar or crumbled white cheese or bleu cheese are my favorites.

VITAMIN B5 – PANTOTHENIC ACID

This is yet another vital B vitamin that can be taken care of with a daily snack on sunflower seed kernels. I will discuss the superfoods in the next chapter. If you want, you can take a 100% RDA supplement like a plain OTC version which is likely fake (which is why I rarely take them.) Otherwise, you should strongly consider covering B5 with sunflower seeds instead.

VITAMIN B6 – PYRIDOXINE

It is important to realize that NATURAL FOOD sources are the way to go. I do eat two 5 ounce cans of tuna fish on occasion as my dinner and ground turkey meat is a main staple of my diet and I eat roughly 8 ounces for dinner at least three nights a week, so four to five nights a week between the turkey and the tuna fish I have taken care of my Vitamin B6 requirements. I have a large supply of most nuts on hand at all times including pistachios, so I can always knock out a cup of them on the nights when dinner will not cover the B6 requirement. In the last chapter I will help you track the vitamins to make sure you are getting everything you need on a daily basis from the foods you eat.

VITAMIN B7 – BIOTIN

Aside from pregnant or nursing mothers, this vitamin is only needed in trace amounts and many natural foods both plant and animal have enough in them to cover our daily requirements. Nevertheless, I do track it and make absolutely certain that it is covered. If you feel that it might be missing in your diet or just want to be sure then by all means you can purchase any B complex and it should be in there as well. Remember that the vast majority of all B complex supplements have the WRONG artificial B12 in them and I will discuss this when we get to it. Since Wheat germ is a must, (2.5 oz. daily) that provides a huge blast of B7 amongst other things like manganese.

VITAMIN B9 – FOLIC ACID or FOLATE

This one is trouble for me. Even in my special prep for beef liver I usually do not eat enough to cover it. However, 2.5 oz. of WHEAT GERM will cover Vitamin B9 and is just about the only food that will. I am still searching for a supplement made from natural sources however, so like me you will likely be forced to take a synthetic version if you skip the wheat germ. B2 and B9 are difficult to cover in a varied daily diet, so these are the two you will most likely have to buy and take on a regular basis and I wouldn't blame anyone if they just went all the way and got a B complex, just be sure it does NOT have the artificial cyanocobalamin in it.

VITAMIN B12 – METHYLCOBALAMIN

This is a HUGE PROBLEM to take as a supplement. The vast majority contain the FAKE CYANOCOBALAMIN which I do NOT TRUST. This vitamin plays a major and intricate role in BRAIN

FUNCTION and I do not know if MY BODY is converting ALL of it into the good form before it ends up in my head.

Because beef liver and sardines are loaded with Vitamin B12 in the good and natural forms, I try to make sure that I use these foods to cover my requirements as much as possible, but when I have to take a supplement I make absolutely certain that it contains METHYLCOBALAMIN derived from natural sources. Yes, it is much more expensive than the usual OTC B supplements and it is very difficult to find in a B complex (I am still looking myself.) Most B complex supplements go for the CHEAP cyanocobalamin and this has forced me to buy EACH VITAMIN B independently which is certainly more expensive and time consuming than if someone would just make a DECENT B Complex with the good version of B12 in it.

CHOLINE

I get most of my choline from beef liver, and eggs, but I certainly do not eat these daily. It takes 6 oz. of BEEF LIVER to cover this. 8 oz. of half and half BEEF LIVER AND TURKEY covers about 80% of the RDA. So I STILL have to supplement my choline. One large 7oz. filet of SALMON will hold about 60%. One cup of CHICK PEAS is about 36%. Choline is the most DIFFICULT of the nutrients covered in this book to get in sufficient amounts in your daily diet. I don't mind taking it in a supplement as long as it comes from a natural source. Check the label and make sure it is in the form phosphatidycholine.

VITAMIN C – L-ASCORBIC ACID

You simply cannot get enough of this vitamin. It is SO GOOD for your health and plays a critical role in countless cellular functions throughout the human body including assisting the absorption and function of many of the B vitamins. It is precisely because of this interdependence of so many of the essential nutrients that we need, that I am very leery of taking supplements. We all know that we should take them with meals because the digestive tract literally "gears up" to absorb nutrients during meals. This means that taking the supplements with meals helps the digestive tract absorb a much higher percentage of the contents of the pill than just dumping it into your empty stomach. However, it is suspected that many components of our food act as buffers as well as catalysts in the absorption of essential nutrients as well and this is in fact part of the reason that these nutrients should be taken with a meal.

To wit, Native Americans never suffered from ulcers due to taking willow bark tea which contains salicylic acid or "aspirin" but many people have suffered from stomach problems by taking the pure active ingredient of willow bark tea in a concentrated pill because the REST OF THE CONSTITUENTS of that tea act like buffers and catalysts assisting in the absorption of the active ingredient and they prevent harm to the digestive tract in the process. This is the most compelling argument for getting our nutrients in natural whole foods rather than pills; we have no way of knowing what else in the natural source plays a critical role not only in the absorption of these CORRECT FORMS of the nutrients present in these foods but also how they might interact deeper inside the body with them and play a critical role in their actual functionality as well.

Since the "WRONG WAY" form of Vitamin C makes up half of all manufactured Vitamin C and is a known TOXIN, you must get your supplements derived from natural sources and listing the ingredient as "L-Ascorbic acid" and not simply "ascorbic acid." Since virtually ALL CITRUS fruits are LOADED with Vitamin C and Acerola berries have possibly the highest concentration of any food on Earth, and kiwis and guavas have higher concentrations than citrus as well, there are plenty of opportunities for you to find these fruits and incorporate them into your daily eating regimen. I have fruit for breakfast daily including guavas from my own trees whenever they are available.

VITAMIN D - CHOLECALCIFEROL

You should ONLY TAKE VITAMIN D3: the NATURALLY occurring form. Because this vitamin plays countless critical roles in the human body including proper bone and tooth formation and maintenance, it is critical for everyone to get enough of it and likely shortages of calcium and Vitamin D3 are the main cause of the current epidemic of osteoporosis amongst the elderly in the United States today. You will get all the Vitamin D3 you need if all you do is spend 20 minutes at a time, twice a day in the sun with your face and arms exposed. You cannot wear sunblock because you are blocking the ultraviolet rays which the skin needs in order to manufacture the Vitamin D3 which is why the exposures should be short. You can also limit your exposure to early morning and late afternoon, but since the atmosphere is blocking most of the ultraviolet during these times your exposures at dawn and sunset should be at least 40 minutes each to be effective.

You can take supplements, just be sure that the vitamin in the pill is true D3 a.k.a. cholecalciferol.

VITAMIN E – alpha-TOCOPHEROL

Most nuts are loaded with Vitamin E but the best are almonds; only 3 ounces of almonds and you have knocked out your daily requirement of this important vitamin. Make it 5 oz. and you can take care of your Vitamin B2 requirement as well. It probably won't come as a shock to know that sunflower seed kernels are also loaded with it and since I eat at least a ½ cup and usually a cup of these on a daily basis I know that my Vitamin E is covered. Chronic deficiency in any vitamin I suspect is one of the major causes of heart disease and cancer which are running rampant in the U.S. and many other developed countries worldwide. The B complex vitamins are all wrapped up in proper brain and nerve function as well as the handling of DNA during cell division and Vitamin E plays a key role in preventing DNA mutation making it NUMBER ONE (along with the B complex) in CANCER PREVENTION IN MY BOOK (This book as a matter of fact!)

So if you have not considered having yourself a cup of sunflower seed kernels yet, now is the time to make that choice and get loads of critical vitamins and minerals including one of the most important ones that may help prevent cancer, just by snacking on a ½ cup of sunflower seed kernels each day. I do, for this reason ALONE, and I hope you will too! (No I don't own any stock in sunflower seeds, but I am considering growing them in the coming year.) If you are going to take a supplement just make sure that it is α-tocopherol (alpha.)

VITAMIN K – n-QUINONES

Your body can make some of this essential vitamin and the good bacteria in your digestive tract also make some (K2) that the intestines absorb as well. However, chronic deficiency can be dangerous, just as bad as severe excess. The vitamin has gotten a bad reputation as the one that "causes blood clotting" so people think it causes strokes and some forms of heart attack, but that is unlikely. The most likely causes of these afflictions are poor cardiovascular health from chronic inactivity, in conjunction with high cholesterol, high animal fat, and high manufactured chemical garbage in our daily diets and a lack of Vitamin E which PREVENTS internal blood clotting.

Still, I do NOT recommend taking a Vitamin K supplement at all especially since the three artificial forms (K3, K4 and K5) are KNOWN TOXINS to the human body. Instead, transform your daily food regimen away from eating a majority of SECONDARY FOODS like grains and, beans and starchy roots that must all be cooked in order to make them edible and make the green leafy vegetables the main course and largest part of your daily diet. Just ½ cup of raw spinach will do the trick. And as long as you are making sure that you are getting your Vitamin E in the good form, then you are well on your way to a longer and healthier life.

END OF CHAPTER QUIZ

1. Name the two B vitamins that are difficult to get in sufficient quantities on a daily basis from natural food sources:
    A. B1 and B3
    B. B2 and B9
    C. B3 and B12
    D. All of the above
    Answer: B. B2 and B9 are the most difficult to get in sufficient quantities on a regular daily basis even though they are found in small quantities in a lot of different foods from eggs to various vegetables.

2. Name the two vitamins that are oil soluble and therefore dangerous to take in extreme excess:
   A. Vitamin B1 and K
   2. Vitamin B3 and B9
   C. Vitamin B5 and C
   D. Vitamin A and E
   Answer: D. Vitamin A and E and oil soluble and A in particular should not be taken in excess of the RDA and E should not be taken in excess of about 200 to 250% RDA.
3. The most likely vitamin related cause of strokes is:
   A. Excess Vitamin K
   B. Excess Vitamin A
   C. Deficiency in Vitamin C
   D. Deficiency in Vitamin E
   Answer: D. Deficiency in Vitamin E. If there is a vitamin related cause to strokes, this is the most likely culprit. Not many people eat lots of sunflower seeds or nuts and these are the only ways to get Vitamin E in good quantity and quality, which prevents internal blood clotting.
4. Chronic deficiency in the following could lead to cancer:
   A. Vitamin C
   B. Vitamin B complex
   C. Vitamin E
   D. All of the above.
   Answer: D. All of the above. Vitamin C deficiency is already linked to immune depression which has been linked to allowing cancer to get started and go unchecked. Almost all of the B vitamins play crucial roles in the replication of DNA during cellular division and chronic deficiency could definitely cause damage to DNA which is exactly what cancer is.
   Vitamin E is a known anti-mutagen (prevents damage to DNA) and since most people do not indulge in sunflower seeds or nuts then this is, in my humble opinion, one of the most likely reasons why cancer has become EPIDEMIC in our country.
5. The artificial forms of which vitamin are known to be toxic:
   A. Vitamin B12
   B. Vitamin C
   C. Vitamin K
   D. Both B and C
   Answer: D. Both B and C. Artificial Vitamin C contains 50% of the "wrong way" stereoenantiomer of ascorbic acid which studies have shown to be TOXIC. All artificial forms of Vitamin K (K3, K4 and K5) are KNOWN TOXINS to the human body. The artificial form of B12, cyanocobalamin has no clinical studies proving its toxicity, but virtually EVERYTHING ELSE we cook up in test tubes is POISONOUS, so I just like to stay away from all of that TRASH.

5. Which nutrient is the hardest to get in natural foods and will likely need to be taken as a supplement?
    A. Riboflavin
    B. Choline
    C. Folic acid
    D. All of the above
    Answer: B. Choline. Few foods are rich enough in choline to cover the 100% RDA of it. If you won't eat wheat germ, Folic acid or "Folates" will be trouble for you as well. Vitamin B2, Riboflavin, is also found in most foods, but in low quantities. Almonds are the best way to solve that problem.

6. Which one of the following can cover not one but three of your daily vitamin requirements?
    A. Spinach
    B. Beef liver
    C. Sunflower seeds
    D. Both B and C
    Answer: D. Both B and C. 1 cup of Sunflower seeds takes care of your 100% RDA daily requirements of Vitamins B1, B5 and E. 3 oz. of Beef liver takes care of four of your daily requirements (over 100% RDA) of B2, B7, B9 and B12.

7. The best natural sources of niacin are:
    A. Turkey
    B. Peanuts
    C. Tuna
    D. All of the above
    Answer: D. All of the above. 6 oz. of turkey, a ½ cup of peanuts, or 6 oz. of tuna will cover your daily requirement of Vitamin B3.

8. The following breakfast will solve two of your vitamin requirements for the day:
    A. 1 grapefruit and 1 slice of whole grain wheat toast
    B. 1 bowl of oatmeal and one banana
    C. 1 bowl of cereal with raisins
    D. None of the above
    Answer: A. 1 grapefruit and 1 slice of whole grain wheat toast. The grapefruit solves the Vitamin C requirement, and the slice of whole grain toast solves the Vitamin B7 requirement.

9. One of the richest sources of Vitamin B9 and the easiest to incorporate into our daily diet is:
A. Beef liver
B. Eggs
C. Milk
D. Wheat germ
Answer: D. Wheat germ. It is also loaded with B9 as well as B7 and manganese in a natural and safe form which is otherwise difficult to find in a natural food source.

CHAPTER 6 – GOOD FOODS and BAD FOODS

To conclude a point from the preceding chapters: We DO NOT HAVE TO INVENT FOOD in TEST TUBES: THE WORLD IS STILL CAPABLE OF MAKING ENOUGH FOR EVERYBODY TO EAT. If people are starving it is because of POLITICS AND GREED – PEOPLE ARE LETTING PEOPLE STARVE, not the Earth.

THE GOOD FOODS LIST – PRIMARY FOODS

I provide this kind of a list in volume 1 – Dieting and Losing Weight, but to recap quickly:

1. **RAW EDIBLE VEGETABLES** – Anything that can be eaten raw including all of the green leafy vegetables from lettuce and cabbage and their kin, from celery to carrots, to onions and garlic are all exceptionally healthy foods loaded with nutrients.

2. **FRUITS** – The vast majority are loaded with Vitamin C along with many other essential nutrients and other constituents that are currently being investigated that have a wide range of health benefits (which I cover in Vol.4 – Antioxidants, Fiber and More.)

3. **NUTS** – These are loaded with Vitamin E and many different minerals depending on the type of nut. Although they are high in fat, it is the good kind, polyunsaturated fat, but they still pack a lot of calories and are not the best friend to anyone trying to lose weight.

4. **SEEDS** – Sunflower seeds are the KING of the SEED foods. They are a SUPERFOOD and highly recommended. Pumpkin seeds and pine nuts are also loaded with essential nutrients and are highly recommended as well.

5) **YOGURT** – This is a very healthy alternative to ice cream. I buy it plain and add my own fruits, nuts and seeds to it or sometimes I buy it with the fruits already added.

6) **FISH** – Sardines, salmon, and tuna are all loaded with essential nutrients, but ALL fish are very healthy foods and an excellent source of animal protein and the Omega-3 that our bodies need.

7) **POULTRY** – Chicken and turkey meat (skinned to remove most of the saturated fats) are the second healthiest animal protein you can eat and should be part of a regular daily eating regimen.

8) **FRUIT AND VEGETABLE JUICES** – Replace soda pop and other junk food drinks with these healthy and refreshing alternatives. ALL vegetable juices MUST be the "Low Sodium" versions. These use potassium salts to make them salty rather than sodium salts. Our bodies NEED HUGE quantities of potassium to ensure proper function of the nerve endings especially for muscle activation. Chronic low potassium is likely the number one cause of heart failure which is the number one cause of death in the United States today. Low Sodium vegetable juices usually contain about 34% of the RDA of potassium in about 12 oz. and drinking two such servings per day could SAVE YOUR

HEART and your life.

THE BAD FOODS LIST

1) **PROCESSED FOODS** – Anything in a box or a plastic bag made from processed grain flour and/or laced with artificial flavors, colors, preservatives and so on (See Chapter 1.)

2. **SODA POP** – Most of these nuisances contain NOTHING THAT WAS EVER ALIVE. The mild carbonic acid which gives them their fizz, is NO GOOD FOR YOU OR YOUR DIGESTIVE TRACT and most are laced with artificial colors and flavors. (They don't need preservatives because even the bacteria want no part of them!) Eliminate this GARBAGE from your diet. Drink vegetable and fruit juices instead as well as plenty of water which is the number one liquid ESSENTIAL NUTRIENT you can drink for better health.

3. **CANDY** – This crud is ALL awful. Eat fruits instead. Many are just as sweet as candy but contain FRUCTOSE which is a very healthy form of sugar that your body does need in order to function. Your brain runs on glucose; no sugar = pass out. Ask anyone suffering from hypoglycemia or diabetes and they can tell you about it. Also, fructose must be converted into glucose which SLOWS DOWN its absorption and arrival in the blood stream.

THE SECONDARY FOODS THAT SHOULD BE DRAMATICALLY REDUCED IN A HEALTHY DIET

1) **GRAINS** – Most people think I am a lunatic when I call these BAD FOODS, and they are not totally evil, but anything that has to be cooked in order to become edible is definitely on the SECONDARY FOOD list which means I do not eat them regularly as a group. Foods made from processed grains like flour are a definite PROBLEM and are BAD FOR YOU. I apologize to all of the bakers out there, but bleached processed white flour donuts, pastries and cookies sweetened with processed white sugar, are DEADLY and mess with your liver and I must insist that I am right here. There are a few exceptions to each rule: see the exception list below.

2) **STARCHY ROOTS** – Anything that must be cooked in order to make it edible including potatoes, yucca, malanga, boniato, etc. I know this is bad news for a lot of people and trust me I miss them sorely too, but the TRUTH is that these foods are ALL very HIGH in calories, and while some may bring some essential nutrients, they are simply not enough to justify the trouble they cause to the LIVER. I eat them very sparingly.

3) **BEANS** – And any other vegetable foods that must be cooked in order to make them edible are all on the SECONDARY FOODS list: eat them very sparingly.

THE SECONDARY FOODS (SHOULD BE REDUCED) THAT ARE NOT SO EVIL AS YOU THINK

1) **EGGS** – Maligned for decades since the discovery of the link between cholesterol and heart disease, eggs are NOT going to kill you unless you eat them raw or by the dozen. I have three eggs

over easy for breakfast about once a week. But my cholesterol is under control. If yours is high you should stay away until you have it under control and PLEASE DO NOT TAKE THOSE TERRIBLE DRUGS TO DO IT (See the upcoming volume on "Taking control of your Cholesterol without DRUGS.")

2. **DAIRY** – I realize that this is a SECONDARY FOOD and many people are developing lactose intolerance. This is due mainly to OVERINDULGENCE and its presence in far too great a quantity in the average American diet. I use a little in my coffee and make one café con leche each day, so my daily intake is a little over 1 cup a day of whole milk. Cheeses and even real butter is fine although I prefer the low fat versions of cheeses and margarines. By the way, I know a lot of people that have switched to 2% skim milk or even 1% and 0% (which tastes like white colored water to me.) Do you know the percentage fat content of whole milk? Most people guess 20% to 50% when I ask them this question and I have to laugh. Do you realize that Half and Half has roughly this percentage of fat? "Whole milk" is an advertising term that started when people complained about the fact that the milk had all of the cream removed and then it was pasteurized and homogenized and to them (back then) it tasted like 0% skim milk tastes to me now. Modern "Whole milk" which has had most of the cream removed is about 3% to 5%. They aren't going to leave much in it because they can sell that cream in the form of cheese and butter and Half and Half at a premium.

3) **BEEF** – Often blamed for causing high cholesterol as well, beef is also not nearly as evil as people now believe. Beef is high in many essential nutrients and the only source of some animal amino acids for most people unless they also eat poultry and fish. Beef liver, which is an organ, and not the beef meat, is one of nature's true SUPERFOODS and it is LOADED with vitamins and minerals and is excellent for you (even if it does make me gag.)

4) **PORK** – Yes, this one is a bit high in saturated fat and cholesterol so if you are having issues with your weight or with cholesterol then you should definitely avoid pork until you have that under control. If you never eat it again in life, the Jews will let you into their synagogues and you probably wouldn't miss a beat on your way to a longer and healthier life (so the Jews are on to something here,) but it certainly won't kill you if you eat it sparingly. I have some sliced pink ham in a sandwich or for breakfast about once a month, and pork chops for dinner about once a month.

**SECONDARY FOODS THAT ARE
NOTABLE EXCEPTIONS TO THE RULES**

1) **OATMEAL** – Even though this is a grain and would normally be considered a SECONDARY FOOD (to be eaten very sparingly) OATMEAL happens to be an excellent "curative" or "preventative" food for the heart. Because it promotes heart health, I advise oatmeal as the ONLY cereal to eat for breakfast. I prefer the "old-

fashioned" oats to the "instant" just because the instant has been "messed with" or processed in some way in order to make it instant. True natural oatmeal is the food that is good for your heart and we do not know how much of its effectiveness has been lost by tampering with it to make it instant. And it doesn't matter that much since regular old fashioned oatmeal boils up in about 8 to 12 minutes anyway. I have it at least four times a week.

2. **CHICK PEAS (GARBANZOS)** – A true SECONDARY FOOD by definition that must be cooked in order to be edible (raw chick peas are harder than human teeth, you would literally chip, crack and split your teeth trying to eat them raw!) Nevertheless, cooked chick peas are loaded with nutrients and good to eat although I still hold them down to about once a week.

3) **GREEN PEAS** – Another legume that is loaded with nutrients and OK to eat on occasion.

4) **LENTILS** – These too should be SECONDARY FOODS and eaten in moderation but they do have plenty of nutrients in them as well.

5) **PEANUTS** – Technically legumes and not a form of nut, they are sort of "in-betweeners" because they do have some nut-like properties including the fact that they are loaded with fat and therefore calories. But they do also have high nutrient content as well. Not the dieter's friend but a snack only when you have nothing else to eat such as a peanut butter and honey sandwich can get you through to dinner.

<h2 style="text-align:center">THE SUPERFOODS</h2>

I try to stick to these as much as possible for two reasons: 1) They guarantee that you will get all of the nutrient that your body needs on a daily basis, and 2) Globally, I believe that High Intensity Agriculture and Animal Husbandry have reached the point that most foods are experiencing a drastic reduction in their nutritional content. In other words, all of those oats are growing in long dead moon dust and if they do not get a continual supply of fertilizer, and irrigation they would shrivel up and die quickly. And trace essential nutrients for plants like molybdenum are extremely expensive (molybdenum compounds cost about six times more than the same weight of solid silver) so I know farmers will never apply it until the plants are showing outward symptoms of molybdenum deficiency. Since all plants need trace amounts of it, then it is fair to assume that all plants grown in that dead moon dust are deficient. And because we are first and foremost vegetarians all the way back to our humble evolutionary beginnings, then it should be obvious that we need it too.

Because of this I believe that ALL nutrients, minerals in particular, are now severely diminished in all of our natural foods. Even a 50% reduction from the late 1800's to now would mean the difference between a particular food in a reasonable portion size having enough of a particular nutrient to satisfy the average person's daily requirement and now falling way short of the mark. And this is exactly why I have had to trim most lists of foods when I look up "Foods high in X" because the majority of them list reasonably sized portions and then they say they have 10% of our daily requirement of the nutrient in them. To me this is a waste of time. Should I eat a dozen eggs of a whole bushel of beans during the day? My goal is NOT to get SOME of the nutrient that I need on a daily basis, rather it is to get ALL of the nutrient my body needs on a daily basis. The SUPERFOODS will help assure us that this goal is met with ease.

This book covers the vitamins (and choline which is close to a B vitamin) so I am concentrating on them here, but in the volume on minerals, some of these superfoods will show up again because some contain high quantities of essential minerals in good forms too. Therefore, I will point out that some of these superfoods bring far more than just those nutrients I am listing in this particular book in the series and are very much well worth the effort of being included into your daily eating regimen.

1) **BEEF LIVER** – Yikes! I HATE this stuff. My father used to get cravings for it and I will always be grateful to my mother that she never made us kids eat it! But it is SO loaded up with essential vitamins and minerals that we must try to get it into our daily eating regimen.

To avoid gagging on it I do the following: 1) I buy 1 pound of beef liver at the grocery store and have the butcher put it through the hamburger grinder. 2) I split this into 3 equal portions at the house and throw it into the freezer, (that's 5+ ounces each,) I thaw one with a 1 pound tube of ground turkey meat and mix them together in a bowl with spices (black pepper, garlic – both ground and minced – and cumin) 3) Cook this burger as you like (I add bread crumbs and make meat balls and bake them in the oven, or without the bread crumbs, I brown patties in the fry pan with a little canola oil, then simmer the patties in stews, etc.)

The point is that this burger meat is now LOADED with Vitamin A, B2, B7, B9, and B12 coming from the beef liver. Two roughly ¼ pound patties have at least 100% of our daily requirements for A, B7 and B12 in the natural form and most of what we need in B2 and a significant quantity of B9 as well. You can make the meat half ground turkey and half beef liver to reduce the amount you need to eat to get those vitamins in 100% RDA amounts in their natural forms.

2) **SUNFLOWER SEED KERNELS** – I buy the kernels rather than the whole seeds because I don't have all day to fight with them. ½ cup of kernels every day is LOADED with Vitamin B1, B5 and E; enough to satisfy our daily requirements for these vitamins. I snack on them during the day and also load them up in the breakfast oat meal. A great way to make your breakfast oatmeal is as follows: 1) Boil regular oatmeal the minimum amount of time the package

recommends, but 2) With one minute remaining add: raisins, nuts wheat germ and sunflower seed kernels. Tasty alternatives include: craisins (dried cranberries) prunes (LOADED with nutrients and very good for you) almonds, walnuts, chopped brazil nuts, pumpkin seeds, sliced banana, etc. Sweeten with honey. You are getting a MONSTER LOAD of essential nutrients in this bowl. In fact, the oatmeal is the minority constituent when I make it up for breakfast!

3) **SPINACH** – raw or cooked, spinach is a powerhouse of nutrients. I happen to love it which does indeed help and I know a lot of people do not care for it, but you should at least try to sneak some in to your tossed salads. If I have a heavy breakfast like the aforementioned oatmeal, I have a tossed salad for lunch which is half iceberg lettuce (almost zero nutritional value by the way) and half spinach. I throw in skinned cucumbers (the skin is bad for you) onions and green peppers (also very good for you) and drizzle a little home made oil and vinegar dressing on top. 1) 1 cup of light olive oil (you can use the dark first pressed extra virgin, but it has a very strong flavor to me) 2) 1 cup of red wine vinegar (it is both sweet and sour and makes a much better tasting dressing) fresh basil, oregano, cilantro, black pepper, and minced garlic. You can tweak the spices until you achieve a flavor that you like.

4) **SARDINES** – Not the most popular fish on Earth I admit, but they are loaded up with Vitamin B12 which is a MUST for proper BRAIN HEALTH and function which in turns leads to having and being in a PROPER MIND. I firmly believe that Vitamin B12 deficiency is the number one cause of INSANITY in our society today. If people had proper BRAIN nutrition which includes ALL of the vitamins and minerals and other essential nutrients in proper forms and amounts, I think everything from pettiness, to fear to crime would all go down. I get sardines in those flat pop top cans plain and add my own mustard or hot sauce even though they do sell them in those sauces. I just prefer my own because I know they are not laced with everything from artificial this, that, and the other or hydrogenated soy which is a DOUBLE WHAMMY EVIL. (Soy by-products are under scrutiny and suspected of being BAD for you, and partially hydrogenated ANYTHING is BAD for you.)

5) **LAMB** – I wish my grocery store would carry it, but there isn't much call for it in my rather small town. It is nevertheless LOADED with nutrients and possibly the BEST land animal meat as far as nutrient content goes. If you can get it and learn how to cook it, I do envy you and strongly recommend it.

6) **SALMON** – Preferably wild-caught and the reason for this is pretty much the same as for avoiding high-intensity agricultural products: limited supply of nutrients to the end product. Fish raised on farms will almost always have a limited food supply especially in VARIETY. This in turn limits the nutritional value of the meat.

Salmon are a true superfood loaded with many vitamins and well worth including in your daily food regimen.

7) **TUNA** – Did you know that some species of tuna are the largest bony fish on Earth? Some weigh well over a TON. They are also some of the fastest swimmers on earth as well. Tuna is a true superfood loaded with many essential nutrients including the Omega-3 fatty acids which contribute to heart health which puts tuna at the top of my list for that alone. But, it is also loaded with vitamins as well. As much as I love to make tuna fish salad, that is NOT the way to go, because mayonnaise is made from RAW EGG WHITES which BLOCK the absorption of the B vitamins. Since we are eating the tuna for the B vitamins, slathering it in mayo is completely self-defeating. The best solution I have found is to make the tuna fish salad with regular yellow mustard instead of mayo. It sounds like it should taste awful, since the tuna has a very strong flavor and the mustard has an even stronger flavor, but it seems that the two cancel each other out. Give it a try, either I am right or my taste buds are ruined. I am not sure which it is!

8) **WHEAT GERM** – What is this stuff? Plants have a very weird reproductive system. Pollen actually delivers TWO sperm cells to the ovum. One joins the ovum cell and grows into a small plant embryo in the seed, the other also joins the ovum and grows into a "germ mass" rather than a twin embryo. Within the seed, when conditions are favorable, the embryo begins to grow and it grows on the germ mass in order to swell and break out of the seed shell. The germ mass is then equivalent to an egg yolk in animal eggs. It is a SOLID MASS OF PURE NUTRIENTS for the seed embryo to grow on first to begin its life. Wheat germ basically contains almost ALL of the wheat grain's nutrients without all of the rest which is relatively devoid of most nutrients. The reason whole grain wheat bread is nutritious is because the wheat germ was kept in the creation of the whole wheat flour. I would argue that wheat germ is by far the best way to go because it is the pure nugget of nutrients within the wheat grain and should be included in your eating regimen as much as possible. I try to eat it at least four times a week (See Oatmeal, for the way I include it.) For those who are gluten intolerant, you will likely have to stay away from it, but that's not a problem. There are other equally nutritious foods.

ALSO NOTEWORTHY

1) **NUTS and SEEDS** – Most nuts are loaded with Vitamin E and minerals. Each nut usually has a high concentration of a specific mineral. Almonds are the highest in Vitamin E, pistachios are loaded with Vitamin B6 and Brazil nuts are loaded with selenium (a rather hard to find trace mineral that we do need.) I try to include shelled nuts in my daily eating regimen in the form of a trail mix: 1) sunflower seeds (you know you can't go wrong there) 2) Raisins (aside from being sweet, these guys are very nutritious and loaded with iron and chromium) 3) almonds, 4) pistachios, 5) pumpkin

seeds (high in zinc and magnesium) 6) walnuts (high in ALA a form of omega-3,) and 7) Brazil nuts. This is very nutritious but the nuts bring a lot of calories, so we can't rely on them to meet our daily requirements of these essential nutrients unless we are willing to burn off those extra with a good daily aerobics workout. 2) **KIWIS, GUAVAS, ORANGES and GRAPEFRUIT** – Guavas are a bit more difficult to find in the produce section of most grocery stores but Kiwis have become a common main stay in most grocery stores across the land and they are loaded with Vitamin C. Just two average sized kiwis will provide you with at least the average daily requirement of the GOOD NATURAL L-ascorbic acid form of Vitamin C and this is HIGHLY PREFERRED over the manufactured form which is 50% of the BAD "left-handed" TOXIC form of the molecule. An orange or a grapefruit can also get you plenty of this all-important vitamin in its natural and preferred form.

END OF CHAPTER QUIZ

1. Which of the following is NOT a PRIMARY FOOD?
   A. Tomatoes
   B. Turnip greens
   C. Cherries
   D. Corn
   Answer: D. Corn. This is a grain and is a SECONDARY FOOD (must be cooked to become edible) which means it should be GREATLY REDUCED in your daily eating regimen. The other three are excellent healthy PRIMARY FOODS. PRIMARY FOODS (edible raw) should make up the BULK of your daily eating regimen.

2. Which of the following are notable exceptions to the SECONDARY FOOD types (are very healthy and can be eaten regularly because of their health benefits)?
   A. Wheat germ
   B. Oatmeal
   C. Chick peas
   D. All of the above.
   Answer: D. All of the above. Wheat germ is a grain product not included in the notable exceptions because it happens to be a SUPERFOOD! (An EXTREME EXCEPTION.)

3. Which of the following are loaded with essential nutrients rarely found in any other food but they are potentially very FATTENING:
   A. Fruits
   B. Nuts
   C. Dairy products
   D. Both B and C
   Answer: B Nuts. Dairy products are certainly fattening as well unless they are skim or lowfat versions.

Alright, so we know we need all of the vitamins in at least the RDA amounts and preferably much higher when it comes to the water soluble ones including in particular all of the B complex and Vitamin C. But it seems like it will take a LOT of EFFORT to plan meals every day to make sure that we get enough of everything. Not to mention the fact that it sounds expensive and most of the really good foods do not sound very appetizing either. What can we do?

There are 14 vitamins that we must get as regularly as possible, or 13 plus choline if you prefer. And the B vitamins in particular are of GREAT CONCERN because chronic deficiencies will MESS WITH YOUR BRAIN and therefore YOUR MIND and I personally do not want to malnourish myself to the point of going INSANE because of it. I am sure everyone will agree with me that being sick is no fun at all, but still HIGHLY PREFERABLE to going INSANE.

All we have to do then, is list these vitamins (in the next volume I will do the same for the minerals and that book is a REAL MINDBLOWER – you will be SHOCKED to find that most people are suffering from severe chronic deficiencies of ALMOST EVERY ESSENTIAL MINERAL and that is DEADLY) and then list all of the foods that can cover them, then fill in the blanks each day and bingo; you've got them all covered.

Personally, I don't like to eat foods that have 20% of the daily requirement here and 30% there. I don't have time to mess around like that, patching together four and five different foods throughout the day just to make sure I have ONE vitamin covered. Multiply that by 41 (the number of KNOWN essential nutrients) and you will have a wall sized chart for every day of the week. That's about as useless as breasts on a bull, to coin a phrase, because it is totally UNNECESSARY.

KNOCKING MOST OUT WITH THE SUPERFOODS

Let's go down the list and see what can be taken care of quickly, easily, and conveniently with a single portion of a superfood.

1) **VITAMIN A** – At least 1 carrot a day will solve this problem with plenty of the vitamin in a safe and powerful antioxidant form.

2) **VITAMIN B1** – THIAMINE – ½ to 1 cup of sunflower seed kernels solves this problem.

3) **VITAMIN B2** – RIBOFLAVIN – 3 ounces of Beef liver of Lamb will solve this problem. 5oz. almonds will also solve this problem. But I do not want to eat these on a daily basis. So B2 is a PROBLEM vitamin that we will have to track.

4) **VITAMIN B3** – NIACIN – 6 ounces of turkey or chicken, ½ cup of peanuts, or 6 ounces of tuna. I don't want to eat any of these

daily, But there are choices and most days I eat enough of one or the other to cover this vitamin as well.

5) **VITAMIN B5** – PANTOTHENIC ACID – That ½ to 1 cup of sunflower seeds solves this problem too.

6) **VITAMIN B6** – PYRIDOXINE – 6 ounces of turkey, ¾ cup pistachios, 10 ounces of tuna. This is another vitamin we will have to track just to be sure we get enough daily.

7) **VITAMIN B7** – BIOTIN – 3 oz. Beef liver, 1 egg, 3 oz. Salmon, the 2.5 oz. of wheat germ or 1 slice of whole grain bread have enough for most folks. The trouble comes from digestive problems or eating raw egg whites so as long as the MAYONNAISE is eliminated (I REALLY miss it and cheat once in while) then it shouldn't be a problem for most healthy adults.

8) **VITAMIN B9** – FOLIC ACID – 6 oz. beef liver, 1 cup chick peas, 1 cup lentils or 2.5 oz. wheat germ will cover your 100% RDA of Folate. This is another vitamin we will have to track.

9) **VITAMIN B12** – METHYLCOBALAMIN – Get used to REFUSING to eat the ARTIFICIAL manufactured form. Most of these manmade chemicals are TOXINS. I expect this one to turn out to be just as bad as EVERYTHING ELSE we make and put in our foods. Ever wonder why they don't sell most medications over the counter and why you MUST go to a doctor to get the prescription? Because MOST drugs will KILL YOU if you are not careful with them. I believe in natural remedies and MOST of those dangerous drugs were discovered in ethnic holistic treatments in the first place and they are FAR SAFER and HEALTHIER for you in those forms. Just 1 oz. of Beef liver has 3 TIMES the RDA, and 3 oz. of either sardines or Atlantic mackerel also exceeds the RDA for this vitamin but since I do not plan to eat any of those on a daily basis we will have to track this vitamin as well.

10) **CHOLINE** – 3 oz. Beef liver, or salmon provides about half of the daily requirement and 1 egg about 25%. 1 cup of CHICK PEAS will cover about 36%. We will have to track this one as well.

11) **VITAMIN C** – L-ASCORBIC ACID – Two to three kiwis a day will solve this problem, or one large orange or grapefruit.

12) **VITAMIN D3** - CHOLECALCIFEROL – About two 20 minute exposures of the face and arms to sunlight will resolve this requirement. For those who do not want to spend any time in the sun or who live at the poles: 1Tbsp. Cod liver oil, 3 oz. Salmon or 8 oz. tuna will also cover your daily requirements for this vitamin.

13) **VITAMIN E** – x-TOCOPHEROL – The ½ to 1 cup of sunflower seeds per day resolves this requirement as well.

14) **VITAMIN K** – n-QUINONES – Spinach is number one and includes other important constituents that contribute to good health and it doesn't take very much of it. Put a half cup in your daily salad and you've got Vitamin K covered thoroughly.

So right off the bat we can cover Vitamins A, B1, B5, B7, C, D3, E and K – over HALF of all of the vitamins that you need – EASILY as follows:

DAILY FOODS THAT SOLVE EIGHT OF OUR VITAMIN REQUIREMENTS

1 CARROT = 200% VITAMIN A

½ to 1 cup SUNFLOWER SEED KERNELS = >100% VITAMINS B1, B5, and E

1 slice of WHOLE GRAIN BREAD = >100% VITAMIN B7

1 GRAPEFRUIT = >100% VITAMIN C

40 MINUTES IN THE SUN = ≈100% VITAMIN D3

½ cup SPINACH = >200% VITAMIN K (eat this every other day)

If we take 2.5 oz. WHEAT GERM instead of the bread we get 100% B7 and B9.

AS FOR THE REST OF THEM...

So EIGHT of the fourteen essential VITAMINS are already taken care of quickly, painlessly and easily and now we can concentrate on the other six.

1) **VITAMIN B2** – RIBOFLAVIN – 3 oz. of beef liver or lamb will more than cover this vitamin, but I do not eat either on a daily basis. So for those days when it is not on the menu I eat 5 oz. almonds to make sure I have it covered. You might notice I am eating a lot of seeds and nuts and they bring calories. Luckily I exercise daily and do a lot of gardening which gets me all the sun I need to make my Vitamin D3.

2) **VITAMIN B3** – NIACIN – 6 oz. of Turkey or chicken, ½ cup of peanuts, or 6 oz. of tuna will cover your requirements for this vitamin. I eat ground turkey or chicken three to five nights a week (at least 8 oz.) and can eat 10 oz. of tuna or whole grain bread peanut butter and honey sandwiches on the other days and have gotten into the habit of making sure I have had one or the other source each day. On those rare occasions when it is not covered, I take a NATURAL Niacin supplement.

3) **VITAMIN B6** – PYRIDOXINE – Since my regular turkey or tuna dinners knock this one out. On the other days ¾ cup pistachios or 10 oz. of tuna fish will cover B6.

4) **VITAMIN B9** – FOLIC ACID – It takes a lot more liver than I usually eat in my ground turkey to cover this one, but a cup of chick peas or lentils will also do the trick. Since I eat 2.5 oz wheat germ most mornings in my oatmeal I know I have my Folates taken care of most days of the week.

5) **VITAMIN B12** – METHYLCOBALAMIN – This one is too important to ignore (although they all are really) so when I don't have my ground turkey with ground beef liver in it, or a can of sardines, then I take a NATURAL SOURCE SUPPLEMENT.

6) **CHOLINE** – When I don't have my ground turkey and beef liver mixture for dinner or my 3 eggs breakfast and some chick peas for dinner I take a supplement for this one as well.

REMEMBER TO STICK STRICTLY TO NATURAL SOURCE SUPPLEMENTS which are NOT found in any of the major stores. I was going to list all of the BAD supplements, but I can make this list short and simple: EVERY SINGLE VITAMIN on EVERY SINGLE shelf in EVERY SINGLE store is a MANUFACTURED SYNTHETIC GARBAGE version of the vitamin. You might think that they are "better than nothing" but you would be WRONG. These vitamins are intimately involved in cellular processes in virtually EVERY CELL in your entire body. Ever hear of MAD COW DISEASE? It is caused by the presence of a malformed protein molecule that causes the others around it to collapse: that's what creates the Swiss cheese holes in their brains and any human's brain who eats even the tiniest quantity of those WRONG MOLECULES – it is not even caused by a virus – just a WRONG WAY MOLECULE. And this particular INCORRECT molecule KILLS and it KILLS FAST.

I am not saying that synthetic vitamins will cause mad cow disease. All I AM SAYING is that if man cooked it up in one of his mad scientist Frankenstein laboratories, you can BET MONEY that it will be TOXIC. And you are also DEPRIVING YOUR BODY of the REAL VITAMIN that it needs while eating that POISON – and that is the definition of a DOUBLE WHAMMY that can make you very sick and even KILL.

TRACK THOSE OTHER SIX VITAMINS

If you are going to stick to my recommended natural sources of the first EIGHT essential vitamins which is quick and easy to do, then just write each of the other six down on a sheet of paper and the foods that will take care of them next to them. If you have one of those foods, cross out the vitamins that it covers. If at the end of the day, something hasn't been taken care of, then take the supplement.

BE SURE TO GET ALL OF THOSE B's

Chronic deficiency on any single B vitamin can mess with your brain and therefore you MIND. Deficiencies can cause BAD MOODS, FORGETFULNESS, DEPRESSION, ANXIETY and make a person not care if they are unhealthy and even prefer it! If you have loved ones that fit this description they might be suffering from a chronic deficiency of one or more of the B Vitamins. Try to fix that if you can. Once a person is brought back to proper health and vitality one of the benefits is that they FEEL BETTER, and they are MORE CONTENT and HAPPY and generally prefer to stay that way too. That means they will take up the task of eating properly and watching their nutrients for themselves thereafter.

THANK YOU AND GOD BLESS AND GOOD LUCK AND ABOVE ALL ELSE; TAKE CARE OF YOURSELF (BECAUSE NO ONE ELSE IS GOING TO DO IT!)

REFERENCES
Most information in this book was found at: wikipedia.org, nutritiondata.self.com, myfooddata.com, WebMD, draxe.com, whfoods.com, and the fda.gov and nih.gov. All of these websites are excellent resources and you should check them out.
[1] The data on Vitamin A was found at:
* https://draxe.com/top-10-vitamin-foods/ Retrieved on 07-23-2018
* https://www.myfooddata.com/articles/food-sources-of-vitamin-A.php Retrieved on 07-23-2018
* http://www.whfoods.com/genpage.php?tname=nutrient&dbid=106 Retrieved on 07-23-2018

[2] The data on Vitamin B1 - Thiamine was found at:
* https://draxe.com/thiamine-foods/ Retrieved on 07-23-2018
* https://ods.od.nih.gov/factsheets/Thiamin-HealthProfessional/ Retrieved on 07-23-2018

[3] The data on Vitamin B2 - Riboflavin was found at:
* https://draxe.com/vitamin-b2/ Retrieved on 07-23-2018
* https://www.myfooddata.com/articles/foods-high-in-riboflavin-vitamin-B2.php Retrieved on 07-23-2018
* http://www.whfoods.com/genpage.php?tname=nutrient&dbid=93 Retrieved on 07-23-2018
* https://ods.od.nih.gov/factsheets/Riboflavin-HealthProfessional/ Retrieved on 07-23-2018

[4] The data on Vitamin B3 - Niacin was found at:
* https://draxe.com/niacin-side-effects/ Retrieved on 07-24-2018
* https://www.myfooddata.com/articles/foods-high-in-niacin-vitamin-B3.php Retrieved on 07-24-2018
* http://www.whfoods.com/genpage.php?tname=nutrient&dbid=83 Retrieved on 07-24-2018

[5] The data on Vitamin B5 – Pantothenic acid was found at:
* https://draxe.com/vitamin-b5/ Retrieved on 07-24-2018
* http://www.whfoods.com/genpage.php?tname=nutrient&dbid=87 Retrieved on 07-24-2018
* https://en.wikipedia.org/wiki/Pantothenic_acid Retrieved on 07-24-2018

[6] The data on Vitamin B6 - Pyridoxine was found at:
* https://draxe.com/top-10-vitamin-b6-foods/ Retrieved on 07-24-2018
* http://www.whfoods.com/genpage.php?tname=nutrient&dbid=108 Retrieved on 07-24-2018

[7] The data on Vitamin B7 - Biotin:
* https://draxe.com/biotin-benefits/ Retrieved on 07-24-2018
* https://en.wikipedia.org/wiki/Biotin Retrieved on 07-24-2018

[8] The data on Vitamin B9 – Folic acid was found at:
* https://draxe.com/top-10-vitamin-b9-folate-foods/ Retrieved on 07-24-2018
* http://www.whfoods.com/genpage.php?tname=nutrient&dbid=63 Retrieved on 07-24-2018

[9] The data on Vitamin B12 - Methylcobalamin was found at:
* https://draxe.com/vitamin-b12-benefits/ Retrieved on 07-24-2018
* https://en.wikipedia.org/wiki/Cobalamin Retrieved on 07-24-2018

[10] The data on Choline was found at:
* https://draxe.com/what-is-choline/ Retrieved on 07-24-2018
* http://www.whfoods.com/genpage.php?tname=nutrient&dbid=50 Retrieved on 07-24-2018

[11] The data on Vitamin C was found at:
* https://draxe.com/vitamin-c-benefits/ Retrieved on 07-26-2018
* https://www.myfooddata.com/articles/vitamin-c-foods.php Retrieved on 07-26-2018
* http://www.whfoods.com/genpage.php?tname=nutrient&dbid=109 Retrieved on 07-26-2018

[12] The data on Vitamin D3 - Cholecalciferol was found at:
* https://draxe.com/vitamin-d-deficiency-symptoms/ Retrieved on 07-28-2018
* https://www.myfooddata.com/articles/high-vitamin-D-foods.php Retrieved on 07-28-2018
* http://www.whfoods.com/genpage.php?tname=nutrient&dbid=110 Retrieved on 07-28-2018

[13] The data on Vitamin E – alpha-Tocopherol was found at:
* https://draxe.com/vitamin-e-foods/ Retrieved on 07-28-2018
* https://www.myfooddata.com/articles/vitamin-e-foods.php Retrieved on 07-28-2018
* http://www.whfoods.com/genpage.php?tname=nutrient&dbid=111 Retrieved on 07-28-2018

[14] The data on Vitamin K – n-quinones was found at:
* https://draxe.com/vitamin-k-deficiency/ Retrieved on 07-28-2018
* https://www.myfooddata.com/articles/food-sources-of-vitamin-k.php Retrieved on 07-28-2018
* http://www.whfoods.com/genpage.php?tname=nutrient&dbid=112 Retrieved on 07-28-2018

www.ingramcontent.com/pod-product-compliance
Lightning Source LLC
Chambersburg PA
CBHW061734250726
48657CB00002B/921